Missing Michael

A Mother's Story of Love, Epilepsy, and Perseverance

by
Mary Lou Connolly

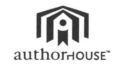
authorHOUSE™

1663 LIBERTY DRIVE, SUITE 200
BLOOMINGTON, INDIANA 47403
(800) 839-8640
WWW.AUTHORHOUSE.COM

First published by AuthorHouse 12/21/05

ISBN: 1-4208-7878-6 (sc)

Library of Congress Control Number: 2005907517

Printed in the United States of America
Bloomington, Indiana

This book is printed on acid-free paper.

In Honor of My Father

This book is dedicated to the anchors of my life: Mom, Barry, Michael, and Meaghan.

Table of Contents

Acknowledgements

I can hardly believe I have written a book and that within its pages, I have exposed part of my family's soul, the place where we live. I am grateful that they allowed me to do so and am appreciative of so many others as well.

Thank you to the dedicated medical professionals who have cared for Michael and the rest of the family throughout the years but most especially to Dr. Sarita Eastman for your unsurpassed caring, Dr. Mark Nespeca for being there whenever we needed you, and Dr. Evelyn Tecoma for your kindness and ongoing commitment to making the lives of those with epilepsy better. We were in profoundly good hands with all of you.

To the educators who stood head and shoulders above the rest: Thank you, Drs. Stewart Seaward and Richard Kelly. You were principals with uncommon principles. May you have many years of happy retirement.

To Madeline Falcone: You are surely an angel in disguise and your coaches are following in your remarkable footsteps.

To the staff and board members of the Epilepsy Foundation of San Diego: Thank you for all that you accomplish with so little and for being there in so many ways, so many times. To Sarah, Jim, Sue, and Steve: Your courage and dedication have been inspirational.

Thanks to Vicky Bennett for suggesting I skip the query letter, agent, and rejection cycle and go straight to AuthorHouse.

To Carmela and Cristina: Thank you for keeping the faith when I didn't.

To Sandy: Thank you for your thoughtful review. I'm sorry you cried, but that's when I knew I might be onto something.

To my girlfriends, without whom I could not have maintained at least some semblance of sanity during various crises: Thank you Anna, Suzanne, Dawn, and Nancy. I'm so grateful you are a part of my life.

To my brothers: Thank you for your support, prayers, and for keeping in touch.

To Barry and Meaghan: Thank you for your love, support, understanding, PATIENCE, encouragement, and trust.

I'm so grateful to my father for instilling within me a love of the written word.

Finally, thank you to Michael: For all that you are and all that you will be.

Foreword

I went public about my son Michael's epilepsy and our family's struggle coping with his often uncontrolled and frequently frightening condition during the fall of 2000. Unable to resist the request of Michael's neurologist, I agreed to participate in the San Diego Epilepsy Foundation's fall fundraiser. It seemed easy enough…I would be a team leader of a bike team. I would only have to ask a maximum of five people to ride. The riders, in turn, would obtain pledges of $150.00 each for sponsorship, and voila, commitment fulfilled.

I dutifully attended the kick-off meeting for team leaders. About twenty individuals designated as leaders were being spurred into action by the rah-rah antics of the event's team coordinator. The coordinator, complete with makeshift halo and angel wings, was unabashed in relating her superior fundraising capabilities; basically, challenging one and all to top her and win a Caribbean trip. I listened intently as I inwardly fought the urge to race from the Coronado Public Library and not look back. Did I really want this bossy, earthly "angel" in my life? I stayed…for Michael, for Dr. Nespeca, and, as I would come to realize later, for me.

I lost out to the angel by mere dollars, raising over $8,000 for the San Diego Epilepsy Foundation. My personal letter to potential donors condensed the story of Michael's ten-year seizure disorder to a page and a half. It was a painful, revealing process to compose that letter. For the first time since his diagnosis, we were letting many people, including some family members, know how profoundly Michael's condition had impacted his life. Until that time, Michael's seizures were mentioned only in passing and almost always after Michael had made it through some crisis. Now, I think of that letter as a beginning and this book as a continuation, of an effort to raise awareness about epilepsy through sharing our personal story including many raw and sometimes discomforting emotions. While writing this book, I have revisited various feelings in recalling specific incidents and I have deliberately not sanitized my reactions of the moment. Right, wrong, appropriate or not, the emotions are what I experienced at the time: fear, anger, disgust, disbelief, despair, pain, rage, protectiveness...and so much more, as my family navigated the rough course of dealing with Michael's intractable (uncontrolled) epilepsy.

Epilepsy is a neurological condition that affects over two and a half million people in the United States (more than cerebral palsy, multiple sclerosis, and Parkinson's combined). Of that number, over 300,000 are children. There are over 180,000 new cases diagnosed each year. In spite of its prevalence in the population, epilepsy does not receive the level of recognition and understanding of many other disorders. I am not above hoping that one of these days a well-known and admired celebrity will "out" the fact that they have a seizure disorder and do for epilepsy what Katie Couric has done for colon cancer and Michael J. Fox has done for Parkinson's disease. Surely, there are actors, baseball and football players, and perhaps even an influential newscaster or morning show personality who has or loves someone who has epilepsy!

The term epilepsy is generally used when an individual has experienced two or more seizures. Seizures can be a symptom of a variety of diseases or incidents ranging from encephalitis to brain cancer; trauma to the head caused by a fall, birth, or a blow to the head; high fever; electrolyte imbalance; blood sugar irregularity; and the list goes on. There are cases that are labeled idiopathic epilepsy. This term means the cause of the seizures is unknown. There are about thirty different seizure forms including tonic/clonic (formerly called grand mal), absence (formerly called petit mal), myoclonic, infantile, partial, Jacksonian, and nocturnal. When all is said and done, epilepsy is a condition that's full extent is difficult to comprehend and therefore may be potentially easier to dismiss or deride.

A largely unspoken fact about epilepsy is that it does take lives. In my small circle of friends and acquaintances, I know at least a half-dozen people who have lost a sister, brother, son, daughter, wife or husband to seizure complications. Epilepsy also takes *from* lives. It takes days and weeks of alertness and awareness, replacing those states with fog and confusion. It takes sleep from parents who worry they won't hear, and thus won't attend, a violent nocturnal seizure. It steals dignity and independence. It fosters fear, anxiety, ridicule, and isolation. And in our case, at times, it has consumed our lives even as we resisted with all our might

The Epilepsy Foundation of America describes a spectrum of epilepsy severity that uses the terms "uncomplicated, compromised, and devastated." Varying levels of severity can occur in any one individual's case. For example, Michael's epilepsy following his initial diagnosis did not complicate his life beyond experiencing mild medication side effects. Later, however, with the loss of seizure control and the addition of multiple medications and episodes of status epilepticus, Michael's epilepsy could easily be characterized as ranging between the latter two descriptions. There is no one-size-fits-all category when it comes to epilepsy treatment. Nor is there one prescriptive way for a family to cope with a child's epilepsy diagnosis.

Epilepsy has made my family's life chaotic and frightening at times. However, it has also given us a unique perspective about the value of health, love, and family unity. The uncertainty regarding what may lie ahead has made us cognizant and appreciative of life's wondrous small moments. It has brought us together in ways unexpected and delightful. It has made us a strong and determined group as we search for the right combination of medication and other treatment modalities that will enable Michael to experience a full and fulfilling life. We have been supported by the caring and concern of our extended family and friends, some exceptional educators, and several dedicated healthcare providers. Michael has dealt with his epilepsy and its complications with incredible courage and perseverance. I hope the story of his journey up to this point in time may inspire others to persevere as well.

Introduction

The intention of this book is to illustrate, through a mother's perspective, the impact of epilepsy upon one family—our lives, our love for one another, our dreams both dashed and realized, our heartache, and our joy. This story does not encompass the whole of our lives nor is there the intent to fully reveal all the particulars of any of our personalities. Rather, the individuals who are described are portrayed in relation to how we acted and how others interacted with us as we dealt with the issues brought upon by Michael's seizures, medications, and associated behavioral and learning difficulties.

This book is not a prescription for how to deal with epilepsy, nor is it a tutorial on the variety of seizure disorders, medications, or other epilepsy treatments. It is merely a recounting of my family's experience in living with this condition for the past fifteen years.

Our experience, because Michael has intractable or uncontrolled epilepsy, is atypical if one believes, as most of the literature suggests, that seventy percent of those diagnosed with epilepsy have the condition controlled through medication. Presumably, most of those individuals go on to lead what are usually referred to as "normal lives." I can assure you that our lives have been a lot of things, but normal...not.

I am a certified white-knuckle flyer. I liken my family's living-with-epilepsy experience to how I feel during a turbulent plane ride. I experience fear and body-numbing terror as the bumps occur, all the while quietly and frantically reciting the Act of Contrition from my childhood. Then, when the ride suddenly becomes smoother, I loosen my grip on the armrests, take a deep breath, and experience the feeling returning to my digits and limbs. And... I wait in anticipation of the next series of bumps. I TRY to look relaxed and normal as I resume conversing with the individual seated beside me. I TRY to engage in and enjoy the smoothness of the ride. I TRY to put the dreaded inevitability of more turbulence aside.

I do not know what the future holds for Michael, the status of his epilepsy, or for the rest of us. I CAN say that I knew instinctively when I came to the "end" of this story, even though I am well aware our lives have many more chapters to be written. I know we will approach them with the love, tenacity, and strength that have brought us to this point. That is the best we can do.

"Making the decision to have a child—it's momentous. It is to decide forever to have your heart go walking around outside of your body." —*Elizabeth Stone*

In the Beginning

Michael Patrick Connolly entered the world on December 5, 1984. His birth by scheduled C-section was calmer than his older sister Meaghan's emergency Cesarean due to a dropping heart rate. All was deemed well in the OR suite when the family pediatrician, Dr. Eastman, remarked, "It's another beautiful Connolly baby." At 6 pounds, 13 ounces, Michael weighed in at one pound less than Meaghan's birth weight, but his head was as beautifully round and cheeks almost as chubby as hers. All digits and features were accounted for, suckling instinct was intact, and lungs were apparently quite sound as well.

Michael's early months were similar to those experienced with Meaghan: good, round-the-clock eater; angelic until the age of three weeks, then, colicky first in the early evenings, then stretching into very late nights. This, I was sure, was my comeuppance for being a nonstop colicky baby (according to my mother) for four months. Fortunately, Barry and I were spared the fourth month of suffering in both of our children's cases. Magically, at the age of twelve weeks, the Connolly children settled down to relax and take in the world.

There were many visitors to our household during the first year of Michael's life. Grandparents, great aunts, uncles, cousins, and a few college friends and their families or spouses-to-be had San Diego, California on their travel itineraries.

My mother and father wanted to be present when their second grandchild arrived and always looked forward to visiting the "little princess," as Grampie

Sullivan referred to Meaghan. Their break from the December cold and snow in Massachusetts was an additional bonus for them. They kept big sister entertained and happy while Michael and I were in the hospital and Barry continued to work. An added benefit of their stay was their help in decorating the house for Christmas.

Christmas 1984 was a festive affair. We were spending our first Christmas in the home we had purchased the previous spring. Barry and I had begun having a Christmas Eve Open House for Meaghan's first Christmas in 1981. Our thought at the time was to gather together any couples we knew who didn't have extended family nearby. In 1981, we had four adults and two children as our guests. By Michael's first Christmas, the guest list had expanded to about forty and included our new neighbors, friends, and their extended family members! Michael was warmly welcomed by this eclectic gathering of those who would become our dearest friends and prime support system in future years.

Michael's first illness, a nasty ear infection, occurred at the young age of three weeks. He was placed on a pink liquid antibiotic that would become somewhat of a staple for him, as he would have several more ear infections prior to the age of six months.

When Michael was three months old, I returned to my part-time job as a discharge-coordinating nurse at the medical center. Leaving an infant at home with a sitter was a new experience for me. The fact that Michael was still breastfeeding complicated matters as well, but a handy manual breast pump and understanding female coworkers who had all done the same, made the transition back to work easier. In addition, I was comfortable with our caregiver choice, Veronica, since our search for her was led by Bill, our neighbor and the prosecuting attorney father of Kristen, who would be cared for by Veronica, too. Veronica's employment interview was conducted a little like I imagined an interrogation would be handled. Nonetheless, she happily accepted our joint offer to care for our children in weekly alternating houses. Veronica proved dependable, caring, and competent and remained in both families' employ until Michael was close to a year old.

During a routine physical check when Michael was about five months old, the pediatrician noted that Michael was tongue-tied. This lay term means that the membrane attaching Michael's tongue to the floor of his mouth extended so far forward he could only stick his tongue out just past his lips. He would need to undergo surgery to clip this membrane. At six months of age, he was scheduled to have his tongue freed. During the same surgery, tubes would be placed in his ears in an attempt to promote drainage and decrease his susceptibility to recurrent ear infections. My experiences in healthcare did not allow me to view these procedures as minor surgery. Counting on guidance provided by my pediatrician friend, Suzanne, I requested that a specific anesthesiologist be assigned to Michael's case. I then received assurance from the director of nursing at Children's Hospital, who was an acquaintance, that both the surgeon and the anesthesiologist had stellar records. On the day of the surgery, the anesthesiologist scooped a smiling Michael out of my arms and promised to return him safe and sound. Barry and I fretted and worried for what seemed like hours but, in reality, was less than one. Our son was returned to us tongue unhinged and ears, presumably, in better shape.

Life returned to normal, the key exception being that Michael absolutely refused to breastfeed from that point forward. So, instead of a weaning process that took three months with Meaghan and culminated in successful drinking from a cup at nine months, we engaged in a significantly more painful cold turkey withdrawal method. At the time, I felt gypped of some nice moments with Michael, but I was hopeful that the surgery which so rudely halted precious nursing sessions would result in fewer ear infections and less time in the pediatrician's office.

In the summer of 1985, Michael experienced his first cross-country plane trip. His big sister was an old hand at this annual excursion to visit East Coast relatives. This was her fourth time. This time, we would introduce the newest Connolly to the large extended family of Sullivans and McCarthys in Western Massachusetts and to the smaller Connolly and Geoghegan units in Boston and Cape Cod.

The trip began with our arrival in Atlanta to attend my brother Brian's wedding to the beautiful Southern belle, Barbara, who won his heart when he witnessed her gritty battle and subsequent win over leukemia. Their marriage was a celebration of life. I hoped throughout the ceremony and for years afterward that I was not witnessing a real-life version of the movie *Love Story*. Throughout rehearsal dinner, a very lengthy church service the following morning, and the reception which followed, a laughing and smiling Michael was passed among loving relatives. He seemed extremely content with his lot in life while his sister danced the evening away with her Grampie and Dad. Barry's mom and his aunts, Kae and Anne, attended as well, so the special introductory visit got underway before we hit the coast.

After our arrival in Massachusetts, in order to reassure grandparents and particularly the paternal great aunts that Michael wouldn't be condemned to the now nonexistent Limbo, we had Michael baptized. In the Catholic faith, baptisms generally occur several weeks after birth, so the sight of nearly nine-month-old Michael jabbering and eating his Cheerios out of a baggie during his group baptism at Sacred Heart Church in Springfield was really something to behold. The aunts were dismayed we had waited so long but relieved that at last, Michael eked out of Limbo danger. The priest, whose altar was littered with cereal, was probably less pleased.

Following the baptism ceremony, Connollys, Geoghegans, Sullivans, McCarthys, and assorted neighbors and friends gathered in my parents' yard for food, drink, and the simple enjoyment of one another. The baptism was the excuse *this* year, though my mom held a similar gathering that Barry called "the showing" each time we traveled east.

This summer marked Grandfather Joe Connolly's eightieth birthday. Mary, my mother-in-law, held a large picnic-style party at White Horse Beach, the location of their beach cottage since Barry's brother Kevin was a baby. Several Sullivans were added to the guest list of beach friends whom the Connollys had known for over forty years. Michael was held and cooed to by a host of beach people during Joe's party. He happily went to just about anyone, which was fortunate, since Joe Connolly had a lot of well wishers who really liked holding babies.

Our trip was filled with love, laughter, and good times as usual. And, as usual, I was teary-eyed and sad leaving all our extended loved ones as we boarded our plane in Hartford, Connecticut. We knew, though, that in a few months, Grammies, Grampies, Grandmothers, brothers, and aunts would visit our small Del Mar home and bunk in Michael's dual-purpose room.

Contrary to our plans and hopes, Michael's propensity for hosting ear infections continued. Just days prior to Christmas in 1985, Michael had what appeared to be a typical cold with a thick, milky nasal discharge. He also had a fever so we were once again on the "sick side" of the pediatrician's office suite. Michael was examined by his regular pediatrician's partner. His temperature reading was 104 degrees. We were instructed to return home and use tepid baths and Tylenol to bring the temperature down. Other than his running nose, Michael played, laughed, and seemed to be very much his pleasant little self.

After dinner, I was playing with Michael on the family room floor when he suddenly went stiff in my arms, his eyes rolling back in his head. I screamed for Barry and we watched with horror as our beautiful baby writhed, turned blue, and began foaming from his mouth. Frantic, Barry called 911 and while I screamed in the background that Michael was not breathing, the operator calmly instructed us to turn his head to one side and protect him from hitting any hard objects. After what seemed like an eternity, he took a gurgling, horrible, but at the same time, sweet-sounding breath, as his limbs spasmed in what would become to us, the all too familiar clonic movements that follow the stiffening ones of a tonic-clonic (grand mal) seizure episode. There was quite a stir that evening in the neighborhood as fire trucks and an ambulance arrived at our home. The firemen and EMTs were wonderfully kind and gentle, and I held Michael in my arms as we traveled to the hospital in the ambulance.

In the emergency room, a very alert Michael was placed in a stainless steel basin filled with tepid water. He looked like one of those Anne Geddes photography babies, all chunky and wrinkled with a head full of curly dark hair and an impish grin. But, Anne Geddes's babies don't have to have spinal taps. Once all of our tears had dried and Michael's status seemed stabilized, we returned home.

I can still picture Barry's face as it looked later that night. Michael was sleeping peacefully and Barry and I were doing our own things to deal with the prior several hours: he, putting together a toy for Christmas at the workbench in the garage, focusing ever so intently on each screw and groove. I was cursing and crying intermittently, cursing the pediatrician because he didn't somehow prevent this from happening nor provide any advance warning it MIGHT happen, and crying because I was wracked with guilt. Why had I dressed Michael in that flannel, zippered, stupid, tan-colored sleeper instead of just a diaper and little shirt so his temperature would not rise so quickly? What was I thinking? What a dope...I should've known better. What the hell good was it that I was a nurse? It was many years before I could view that pediatrician in a positive light...knowing that certainly he was not to blame. Self-forgiveness would take time as well...maybe never completely. For Barry, the evening's event was the start of a thinking process about not wanting to face another similar episode. The culmination of his emotional upheaval was a decision to have a vasectomy the following year.

The following day, a large vase of flowers was delivered with a beautiful message stating that our neighbors and friends, Anna and Don, would be there for us whenever needed. They had whisked Meaghan to their home the evening before when the fire engines and ambulance arrived. I pretty much dissolved when I read the card and later that day, nearly melted down when Don wrapped me in a gentle bear hug and verbalized what the florist had written. Over the years, for too many to think about, I would keep such emotions wrapped pretty tightly, fearful that showing them would somehow validate the sometimes horror we were living.

We were instructed in the emergency room to be very cautious about controlling infections and fevers for several years, since children with one febrile seizure are prone to reoccurrence until the age of five when the seizure threshold supposedly increases. We worked diligently to put the trauma of the seizure behind us and focus on the many delightful aspects of our life: we had each other, great jobs at solid companies with good benefits, we lived in a lovely home in a vacation paradise, and had two beautiful children and loving family and friends. We would overcome this blip on our otherwise unblemished American Dream life.

"The force of the waves is in their perseverance." —*Stephanie Luetkehaus*

Speaking of Barry...

Some people are lucky in love and I count myself among them. Of course, I really don't believe luck has very much to do with the art of finding and keeping a suitable mate. Common interests, mutual life goals, and an appreciation for the complementary traits of the other partner go a long way toward developing a solid relationship. To paraphrase that handsome, famous sports agent, completing one another is a pretty successful formula.

The man who would be Michael's father was born and raised in Brookline, Massachusetts, the second son of Mary and Joe Connolly. At the age of twenty-six, when we first met, he was living in the same home where he grew up. Barry's upbringing with two spinster aunts occupying the same home gave him a unique, humorous, and tolerant view of life.

Barry attended Rensselaer Polytechnic Institute, an engineering school in New York State, where older brother Kevin had paved the way. Apparently, it wasn't all about studying, and that would become clear during an alumni weekend when I accompanied Barry to his old frat house. College friends eagerly told the new girlfriend about the various escapades of "The Admiral," Barry's moniker due to his Navy ROTC membership. Never one to back away from a party or fun time, I was nonetheless pleased that I met Barry at another time in his life. He served in the Mediterranean Naval fleet during the Vietnam era. He ended his tour as a young officer with a little less love for ships but, thankfully, he was intact and ready to pursue a graduate education at Boston University.

The fateful night occurred in July 1973. I had just graduated from Boston College. My roommates Mary Lee and Lynn gave me an instamatic camera as a gift. I took it on our celebration cruise of Boston Harbor, which was sponsored by a favorite hangout called Copperfield's. While on the cruise, I noted a guy who intrigued me only because I couldn't imagine how he could see to navigate the downward stairs through the thick mass of dark brown curls that covered his eyes. Later in Copperfield's, I found myself standing next to the curly-haired one. I proceeded to take his picture…flash…from about a six-inch distance, and as I am quite fond of saying, he's been blinded ever since.

A courtship followed wherein the Red Sox, Celtic, and Bruin games were the date venues of choice. After we went together for about six weeks, I announced to my roommates, "This is the guy!" I was really comfortable with him and thought he was the perfect partner. They looked at me as if I'd really lost it. They knew Barry by then and to them, he did not appear to be soon-to-be married material. They were right. Imagine my surprise when a year later, the subject of marriage came up during a chance meeting with one of my coworkers. Barry's reply slipped out quite easily…"I'm never getting married." Oops. This was going to be tough. It would be almost four more years before the ultimate commitment would be made. I can rightly say that Barry never proposed marriage, he merely caved.

My parents felt good about Barry from the first meeting. I brought him home to Western Massachusetts with me after dating him for only a few months. The ruse I used to have him accompany me was that my first car, a Chevy Vega I had named "Babs," was acting up and I didn't want to chance a breakdown alone on the Massachusetts Turnpike. Babs made it. We arrived at the El Paso Street address on schedule. My mother's first remark when Barry was out of earshot was "He reminds me of your father." I thought that was an especially good sign. My father, I think, especially appreciated Barry's quiet and accepting demeanor. He also appreciated the fact that Barry wasn't at all like my prior boyfriends. Barry, as it turned out, could do no wrong in either of my parent's eyes.

We were married in April 1977. For a guy who resisted for so long, marriage was a remarkably easy adjustment. We settled in Dearborn, Michigan where Barry had lived since 1975 when he was hired out of graduate school by Ford Motor Company as a financial analyst. He had made many friends there prior to our marriage. They were a close, fun crowd and most were single men. The guys—Mike, Eddie, Terry, and others—were very accepting of a new mate, so we joined in the singles fun of disco clubs, enjoying new restaurants, and trips to the Kentucky Derby and other major horse races. We were always the dependable double date when one of the guys needed us.

Barry recognized that the auto industry was ready for a downturn in 1979 and suggested we move west. I was game. Though I liked my job as a home care administrator in Ann Arbor, it was a thirty-five-mile drive one way, and many days, the drive was hampered by hazy fog, black ice, or blinding snowstorms. We were both tiring of the grayness of Michigan weather and the sameness of the two seasons: winter for nine months and three months of simmering summer.

We narrowed the West Coast destination down to an area called La Jolla outside of San Diego. Barry had driven through it once on a Navy liberty and he thought it might be nice to settle there. We made a brief reconnaissance trip in August during which we found a great place to live and each of us had a job interview as well.

In a heartbeat, we sold our cars, packed our belongings, and sent them via moving van to our duplex in La Jolla. We treated ourselves to first class seats to San Diego—thanks to a terrific American Airlines promotion. It wasn't exactly what the pioneers of old did, but we felt pretty adventuresome nonetheless when we arrived in California in September of 1979.

What followed was six great months of unintentional unemployment. Our duplex on La Jolla Boulevard was about three blocks from the beautiful Wind and Sea Beach. We had many friends and family members who came to visit California. We took advantage of their visits to experience our new locale as tourists. And though our job searches continued fruitlessly, we had lots of optimism about the future. The situation pretty much epitomized the Barry part of our couple equation…always glass full (we'll get jobs), never reckless (sufficient funds were in savings), contemplative, yet adventuresome.

Our carefree California existence ceased when we received job offers from the companies we interviewed with during our scouting mission. Once we were gainfully employed, we started discussions about having a family. Before doing so, I needed to clarify something with Barry. Though I loved my father-in-law, Joe, I knew that he took little interest in the rearing of his infant and young sons, leaving that to Mary and the aunts. Joe was more into the boys when they could converse at his level. If we were going to have children, I

9

wanted a partner in parenting just as my dad had been. Barry assured me he wanted the same.

Meaghan was born in March of 1981. Barry took to fatherhood as he had to marriage…with enthusiasm, total commitment, and an enormous capacity to love.

"Begin doing what you want to do now. We are not living in eternity. We have only this moment, sparkling like a star in our hand–and melting like a snowflake." —*Marie Beynon Ray*

Blissful Ignorance

Michael's development continued normally during the second year of his life. He walked at a year, was talking appropriately, was full of energy and inquisitiveness, and had a certain impish quality about him. Oftentimes, when I was in public places such as malls or grocery stores, complete strangers would approach me and most would use the same word to describe Michael: "engaging." And that he was.

We did experience that frightful period described as the "terrible twos." For Michael, that period began a few months prior to the official age of two years and lasted a few months after he reached the age of three. It was a time when we stopped going to restaurants because such outings caused immeasurable stress and strain to one or both parents. Even Meaghan, at her young age, could appreciate it would be best to avoid the public display of her brother's demonstration of temper, stubbornness, and horrific tableside manners.

In October, we traveled to my brother Gary's wedding in Washington, D.C. The bride was lovely, the ceremony perfect, and we had a wonderful time seeing the Washington sights. However, each meal, including the rehearsal dinner, the reception, and the day-after wedding brunch for the relatives, was punctuated by Michael's "terrible two" behavior. I look at the pictures that were recorded of that trip and I see a smiling, cherubic, nearly two-year-old looking back at me. "Not the same trip," my mind whispers.

Michael loved to entertain. In these early years, he had not a bit of shyness about singing the newest preschool jingle to a host of relatives and friends.

His repertoire wasn't limited to the nursery school singsongs. He belted out rock tunes especially Springsteen's, and loved to wear a denim jacket and play a pretend guitar while shaking and gyrating to "Born in the USA." This was usually performed while wearing an oversized football jersey that was his nightwear, so it made for a very amusing sight. I was quite convinced during this time period that Michael was destined to be on some kind of stage or, at the very least, involved in activities in which he could optimize his hamming it up and acting abilities.

He loved his preschool and was well behaved and attentive there though mischievous and daring, too. The staff was familiar with me since Meaghan had also attended, so several of the teachers were there to greet me at the end of Michael's first day. They could hardly wait to report, while suppressing giggles, that Michael and another boy named Marsh decided to see whose pee could go the furthest in the school's sandbox area. This act, I guessed, was the forerunner of the adult-version pissing contest. I thought this was fairly normal, amusing, and another indication that I indeed had birthed a boy.

Michael was equally comfortable, fun loving, and talkative with family, adults, and children of all ages during these formative years. He was amusing, bright, cheerful, and energetic. He was a hit with teachers, doctors, sitters, and others entrusted to care for him. He was very loving toward and tremendously enjoyed by all of his grandparents and delighted them in return. In fact, he seemed particularly attached to the elder people in his life.

We continued to take our annual vacations to Massachusetts, dividing our time between Western Massachusetts and Cape Cod. My family had an open invitation to stay at the Connolly beach cottage; so most days were filled with one adult or another taking the kids walking on the beach, shell collecting, or exploring the sandbar. Many days, the entire troop of adults and children would venture off to the Marshfield Fairgrounds where Grandfather Joe could play the horses and the younger ones could examine the sheep, goats, and fair food. The crowded cottage filled with Connollys, Geoghegans, Sullivans, and assorted friends, spouses, and wannabe spouses, was a joyous celebration of family and fun that we all looked forward to each year.

During Michael's first five years, the most serious health problem continued to be his chronic ear infections. In our day-to-day family operations, the most visible sign of that issue occurred during daily baths when we gingerly washed hair around earplugs, and tried to ensure that sibling bathing time didn't result in undue errant splashes. Memories of Michael's febrile seizure caused us to be extremely vigilant about reporting each and every sign of a cold or potential infection to the pediatrician.

Michael's second set of ear tubes was placed at eighteen months of age and they came out spontaneously at age three. We chose not to have another set placed, hoping that instead, he was outgrowing the problem.

Ear infections aside, Michael's development in the first five years was on par with his sister's. We did not observe any lags as there often are with boys. He was potty trained at just over three years of age in spite of a disastrous attempt on my part to implement the concept of potty training in a day. After several hours of trying techniques in a book recommended by the pediatrician, my only results were extreme frustration on my part and recognition that my son had quite a stubborn streak. Feeling horrible for putting us both through the experience, I pitched the book and let the headstrong child have his way a few more days. Then one morning, I announced nonchalantly that I had forgotten to buy diapers. That day, our official training commenced and was completed!

In February of 1989, we were preparing to move to a house about three blocks from our first home. A week before the moving date, our home was broken into while we were away at work. We had experienced another burglary several months earlier, which I interrupted upon returning from work. In the previous break-in, stolen items were limited to several sentimental pieces of jewelry and our stereo unit. In the second instance, we had unwittingly assisted the thieves by having most of our belongings packed in boxes and ready to go in preparation for our move. Though the experience at the time was extremely traumatic and frightening, my memory of entering our home that evening brings a smile to my face. Upon opening the front door in a state of panic caused by seeing two police cars with their bubbles on outside the house, I saw Michael following and mimicking one of the younger officers as he excitedly told me he was "helping the cop" fingerprint the area.

Minus many of our possessions, we moved into our new home the following week assisted by neighbors and friends. Since we were remodeling the upstairs of the house, for several weeks, the four of us slept together on mattresses lined up across the downstairs family room. Nights were peaceful in spite of the crowded, shared conditions.

We were all very happy in our new environment. We had twice as much room, yet remained by our neighborhood friends. We could keep the children in a school system with an outstanding reputation. We would have a security system installed in this home. We had excellent daycare, preschool, and after-school arrangements. We had good jobs, schedules that were family-friendly, and as I liked to note, a lap for each child. In a nutshell…life was good!

"We relish news of our heroes, forgetting that we are extraordinary to somebody, too." —*Helen Hayes*

Back to Meaghan

Meaghan was born about 4:30 a.m. on March 21, 1981. She had stubbornly refused to budge from the womb the previous day when I was sent home from the labor suite dejected that I had falsely identified the not very painful cramping in my abdomen as labor. No wonder I had remarked to Barry on the way to the hospital that the pains "weren't bad at all." I couldn't understand what all the fuss was about. Well...the very next day I understood perfectly well, and when Meaghan's heart rate took a dramatic drop and I received an epidural for the impending C-section, I was relieved to be rid of the pain and concentrate on the birth of a healthy baby.

She was the cutest infant I had ever seen. I was certain anyone looking in the nursery and talking about how beautiful a baby was, most definitely was focusing on the bassinet that read "Meaghan Fitzgerald Connolly." We marveled at her perfection: rounded head, cute little nose (thankfully, like Barry's), teeny little ears nice and close to her head (whew, no Sullivan ears), curious dark eyes, and the chunkiest pink cheeks. We could hardly bear not to look at her—this wonder we had created. When Meaghan was six or seven weeks old, we were sitting at our usual weekend spot on a remote area of Wind and Sea Beach in La Jolla. The woman who lived on the property above the beach approached us. She told us that she and her husband had so enjoyed the last several weekends as they watched the couple that couldn't seem to stop themselves from constantly looking in the baby buggy. She just had to come and get a look herself!

Meaghan was not just the apple of her parents' eyes. She was the first Sullivan grandchild, and had frequent visits from her doting grandparents and besotted young uncles. She was the second Connolly grandchild and the first girl, so she was greeted as a bit of a novelty by Grandmother and the Nanas, Kae and Anne.

Grandfather Joe would have to wait for Meaghan to make the trip east. A bout with Guillain-Barre Syndrome following a swine flu injection, left him rehabilitating weakened legs that had been paralyzed for several weeks. His goal, he told us, was to be using "just a cane" by the time we got to White Horse Beach in the summer. He would meet that goal, of course, and then some. The cane was discarded during our August visit and the man who really wasn't much for babies, held his granddaughter plenty in his still weakened arms.

When Meaghan was about sixteen months old, Barry made a rare tactical error regarding his career. Unhappy at the company that had employed him for two years, he chose to quit just prior to our annual trek to the East Coast. His plan was to begin job hunting when we returned. Naturally a worrier, I was calmed by Barry's optimism and focused on observing assorted relatives enjoy our walking and talking, petite, dainty toddler.

Unfortunately, the job search continued until the following summer. I resisted going back to work for many months since I was thoroughly enjoying my time at home with Meaghan. Diminishing savings and a yearning to own a home some day forced my hand. I took a part-time job with a local nursing registry performing their payroll and placement functions. I hated the job. It was dull, boring, and made ill use of any of my skills. Therefore, I jumped at an opportunity to consult at the medical center when requested by Sonya, a friend who had been my boss in Boston and had relocated to San Diego. I had just accepted that job when Barry learned he had been hired at one of the local aerospace businesses. A nearby daycare provider was located for Meaghan, and she quickly adapted to spending part of her day with a few other children and a squawking parrot.

Several months later, we purchased our first home in nearby Del Mar. Meaghan's playgroup friend since birth, Katharine Tremblay, lived across the street. The three-year-olds delighted in one another's company. The families formed a lifelong bond that would provide strength and support in the years to come.

Meaghan attended Del Mar Hills Preschool, a remarkable place that managed to combine sufficient unstructured play with Montessori and an innovative musical program. Ursula, Regina, and the well-prepared teachers who worked for them, provided an enlightened environment that supported learning and social development. Meaghan flourished.

It was during these preschool years that Grammie Sullivan used to worry out loud that the world would take advantage of Meaghan because she was so sweet and trusting. It was a grossly unjustified concern.

Meaghan attended the local grammar school around the corner and made friends that would be her companions throughout high school and into college. She joined a Brownie troop and several weeks into it decided Brownies were not for her. I was delighted. At least I could scratch "Brownie mom" off my list. She played recreational soccer and demonstrated particular competitiveness when part of a mixed-gender indoor league. She danced for a few years…ballet, tap, and jazz…alongside Katharine and Katharine's younger sister, Jacqueline. The experience of transforming innocent-looking young girls into stage-ready nymphets was far different from the Irish tap dancing of my youth. When presented with a choice between dance and soccer, Meaghan chose soccer. Yea!

During Meaghan's childhood, we did our best to shield her from any concerns we had about Michael's health. That became an impossibility during her junior high and high school years, as his condition was undeniable when medications were not working and stays at Children's Hospital impacted everyone's lives.

Meaghan has always been a fierce advocate for Michael, yet never let him get away with anything simply because he had epilepsy or was getting used to one medication or another. Whenever Michael was in the hospital or going through a difficult medication adjustment, Barry and I were careful to give Meaghan her special time with us. It must be a mixed bag of emotions for the sibling of a child with a chronic health condition. That being said, the majority of the time, Meaghan reacted to her younger brother in the same manner as most older sisters. She was appropriately protective, often annoyed, many times impatient, and frequently caring.

Though I was well aware of my daughter's inner strength and her capacity to learn from and adapt to most situations, there were still circumstances when I would observe her with a mix of astonishment and admiration. When we visited the Connolly household in the summer of 1993, Barry's mother was severely incapacitated by a precipitous neurological condition. The shock was evident in Meaghan's face as she hugged her drooling, hard-to-understand grandmother....she who had stood laughing and joking in our California kitchen just a few months earlier. Soon, thereafter, Meaghan brought out her manicure kit and gave her grandmother the complete salon treatment. She did so each day of our stay, giving Mary her undivided attention and the comfort of her gentle touch. She interacted with Mary with skill and grace beyond her years. When Mary died the following spring, Meaghan mourned, but was grateful her grandmother was at peace.

The next personal loss would be a sudden one occurring in 1995 just prior to Meaghan's fourteenth birthday. When my father succumbed at age sixty-nine to the ravages that a six-week series of strokes had caused, Meaghan had great difficulty knowing she would not see her beloved Grampie again.

She worked through her grief in a special way. Through her tears, Meaghan prepared a beautiful album about her grandfather, filling it with quotations she felt captured his essence, and with photographs that portrayed him as son, husband, fire chief, father, grandfather, and friend. It is a poignant compilation of a granddaughter's great love, and material evidence of the strength and resilience that lie within her. My mother usually leafs through the album at least once every visit. I pick it up when I'm really missing my dad. It brings him closer than the multitude of picture albums throughout the house. Meaghan really did manage to capture his spirit throughout the loving pages she created.

As she has grown older, Meaghan's strength and integrity have become even more evident. She emerged from the wildly liberal UC Santa Cruz campus with an intact sense of self and harboring a rich mix of liberal and conservative views, beholden to neither radical extreme. Her decision to attend law school was not a surprise. I look forward to her honing her views about ethics, healthcare, justice, and equality and then, making what I know will be a significant mark on the world.

Meaghan...fiercely loyal and strong, belying her petite frame and freckle-faced innocent looks; Meaghan...passionate in her views and beliefs but unwilling to impose them on others; Meaghan...incredibly intuitive and outrageously witty; Meaghan...a tolerant listener without patience for intolerance; Meaghan...still engendering the same parental awe and amazement as she did in her baby buggy.

"Security is mostly a superstition. It does not exist in nature. Life is either a daring adventure or nothing." —*Helen Keller*

Almost Five

Halloween never meant much to me until I met my friend Anna. I could hardly dress my kids as hobos every year when she showed up with her children dressed in elaborate costumes that she, of course, had made herself. I never did master the art of whipping up a Snow White or Musketeer garb on a sewing machine, but I sure did learn to create the most horrific witch, vampire, and monster faces.

On October 31, 1989, Meaghan was a witch for at least the third year in a row, and Michael determined he would be a pirate. Whew! That one I could put together fairly easily. Michael seemed a bit out of sorts that evening. Nevertheless, he got dressed in his costume and joined Anna's children and others for trick or treating in the neighborhood.

Tired and heavy-eyed, he went to bed early. The next morning, I noted the spot on his chest, and a visit to the pediatrician confirmed that he had the chicken pox. His seemed a mild case; a few pockmarks on his body, a couple on his face and neck. I stayed home with my infectious child, and he seemed to be absolutely fine except for the red spots and developing scabs he had in a few places.

On night nine of the chicken pox episode, Michael complained that the back of his head hurt right about where a scab was evident. He not only complained, he whined and cried, a behavior not consistent with his previous high pain tolerance. I rocked him in my arms for a time, and he settled into what seemed to be a peaceful sleep.

The following morning, Michael was free of complaints and wanted to play with the neighborhood children. Since he was no longer contagious, we allowed him to play in the front yard with his sister and their friends. He was happy, calm, and appeared to be recuperating well from what I considered at the time to be a routine childhood illness.

Later in the afternoon, Barry and I sat reading in the family room, and Michael was busy coloring at the child-sized table adjacent to it. Suddenly, Michael fell from his chair. My immediate thought was that he had pushed himself away from the table carelessly and caused himself to lose balance. It became all too clear only seconds later, that we were witnessing another tonic-clonic seizure. This time, our almost five-year-old son lay on a hardwood floor, stiffening violently while we watched helpless and terrified. Every feeling of four years ago returned...Is he breathing? Will he choke? How long can this go on? What should we do? After a couple of seemingly endless minutes, the gasp for air and rhythmic jerking of limbs came, then stillness and minimal responsiveness to our pleading screams, "Michael, can you hear us? Michael, it's Mommy...Michael..."

Though we were experienced enough to know that this time we did not need an ambulance, we still ended up bringing Michael to the local emergency room. The on-call pediatrician noted that Michael had no fever, nor did he show any signs of encephalitis. He scheduled Michael to have an electroencephalogram (EEG) the following day.

Barry and I were shaken. Michael seemed just fine. We went about our normal routines pushing aside thoughts that this was more than a one-time occurrence.

Michael and I went to Children's Hospital for the EEG the next day. He threw up the chloral hydrate meant to sedate him, but managed to remain still for the electrode placement and head wrapping with gauze, and to sleep on demand for the EEG anyway. Dr. Eastman informed us several days later that Michael's EEG was normal and no further tests, procedures, or worries were indicated. We breathed.

Ten days after that episode, Michael and I were in my bedroom getting ready for work and pre-school. I remember his outfit—cute Hawaiian shorts and an aqua jersey. He came partly out of my bathroom standing in the door jam. He looked directly at me, then his eyes moved in unison to the right. I knew then, what to expect. I ran to him and laid him on the carpet where his little body could go through the spastic movements of a tonic-clonic seizure without the danger of harming limbs or head. There was no need for paramedics or the emergency room. I looked, I waited, and I sobbed.

I called Dr. Eastman. She was incredulous. "Michael was perfectly normal," she said. "How could he have two seizures in ten days?" she asked me. She ordered a magnetic resonance imaging (MRI) to be done that day. I often thought over the years that Dr. Eastman had almost as much difficulty accepting Michael's diagnosis as we did.

Barry returned from work and the three of us headed to Children's Hospital to rule out the possibility there was something an MRI could detect, that was in Michael's brain causing this dysfunction.

The process of doing a MRI on a child Michael's age involves the administration of anesthesia. It was comforting to me that the anesthesiologist was the same one who administered Michael's anesthesia for his first surgery. The pre-procedure and actual MRI procedure time took several hours. As we paced and sat in the waiting room, Barry and I were imagining the worst possible outcomes and keeping them to ourselves.

Once the MRI was completed and Michael was awakened, we were moved to the day surgery post-operative area. After what seemed like another entire day, the neurologist on-call arrived. The large, rotund, kind man put his arms around me and told me, "Nothing is there, no brain tumor, it's just a seizure disorder."

At that moment, I felt enormous relief. No tumor, not cancer, I won't lose my baby. It's only a seizure disorder. Armed with a Phenobarbital prescription, the three of us left. Clearly, we had not made it to that five-year marker without another seizure. But, our Michael didn't have a brain tumor!

We were anxious to learn all that we could about seizures. I contacted the local Epilepsy Foundation and was supplied with informative and useful material that satisfied our initial need to know. While we were serious about learning all that we could about epilepsy, both Barry and I were certain that Michael would be in the group of children who 1) respond to their medication regimes by having no seizures and 2) discontinue taking medication after two seizure-free years.

"Some of the most important things in life aren't things." —*Linda Ellerbee*

Another Countdown

Michael's initial adjustment to Phenobarbital was disturbing to all of us. He was easily irritated, cranky, and appeared to be easily distracted.

Two weeks into the medication, he broke out in a rash. I tried calling the neurologist, who was now Michael's specialist, to report what I feared was a medication side effect. When two days had passed and my call was not returned, I must admit I lost faith in the kindly man who had given us the no-brain-tumor news.

It turned out Michael had a not uncommon childhood ailment called Fifth's Disease, which we discovered thanks to my friend Suzanne's diagnosis. We were able to keep him on Phenobarbital, but now we were on the lookout for another neurology practice that might return calls more promptly.

Dr. Eastman suggested that we could try another neurologist she knew who saw mostly adults but was willing to take on Michael's case. So, we would be under the care of Dr. Chaplin and were satisfied, I might add, for the next two years.

Michael's preschool teachers at Del Mar Hills Nursery School were understanding and sympathetic regarding his diagnosis. It was not difficult to leave him there under their watchful eyes and within their nurturing environment.

We often found ourselves asking if this or that behavior was the Phenobarbital or was it just a five-year-old boy acting out. We pretty much accepted we didn't or couldn't know and dealt with his unacceptable behaviors the same as we always did. We worked with Michael to change them

Michael's coordination and physical capabilities during these years were not impacted by epilepsy or the medication, so the activities of T-ball and soccer were undertaken. Barry coached Michael's T-ball team for two years. The stands were filled with parents who were amused by the Del Mar team's first two innings of blooper hits, missed catches, and errant throws. The third inning (the last one in a T-ball game) was usually ploddingly slow and ceased to be amusing to just about all spectators.

I remember thinking during those games how lucky Michael was compared to a couple of his teammates who were shuttled between divorced parents and victims of their parents' ongoing disputes. More than a few times, these kids' late arrivals at the field were explained by the delivering parent as the fault of the other parent for not informing them of the schedule. As things turned out, lucky was probably not the description of choice regarding Michael.

Soccer in California can occur pretty much during every season and for us, it did. Michael played with his Del Mar League teammates in the fall and early winter, and in the indoor or "walled" boy/girl league in spring and summer seasons.

Michael's head was definitely in both of these sports. Even at his young age, he knew how to play his position. While not a prolific hitter or goal scorer, he was a smart player and enjoyed his times on both fields of play.

Michael's kindergarten teacher was young and inexperienced but kind, patient, and tuned-in to each of her kindergartner's needs. In Michael's case, her goal was to increase his focus and attentiveness to tasks. By year's end, Mrs. Polarek was satisfied with his progress and confirmed so in Michael's report card and recommendation to proceed to first grade.

First grade brought another young, insightful teacher into our lives. Her students universally loved Mrs. Wheeler with Michael being no exception.

Michael would be seven that December. Delightedly, we noted that he had experienced two seizure-free years. Dr. Chaplin worked out a schedule whereby we were to decrease his Phenobarbital gingerly and, if no untoward effects occurred, we would be "home free."

The initial weeks of lowering the Phenobarbital dose were uneventful with the exception of noting Michael was more alert and less irritable. This was going to be a good thing!

One day, during this withdrawal period, I picked Michael up at the Del Mar Hills Nursery School after-school program for their "graduates." As we walked back to the car, Michael seemed to be in a trance focusing on a metal object on the sidewalk. When I called his name, he responded, but I was uneasy about the occurrence. During the next several days, two or more similar incidents led me to call Dr. Chaplin. He arranged for an EEG in his office.

I could tell that something was really wrong by the look on the EEG tech's face. I absolutely knew it when she said to keep Michael on his current Phenobarbital dose and wait for Dr. Chaplin's call.

An EEG abnormality was confirmed. Dr. Chaplin used the term "absence seizures" and he attempted to continue treatment by increasing Michael's Phenobarbital. Now, it appeared Michael had a more complex condition and Dr. Chaplin, I believed, really wasn't certain he wanted to deal with it. I could understand that. It appeared at this point Michael needed to be followed by a pediatric neurologist familiar with the myriad of seizure disorders that can occur in childhood. We planned to pursue a change of physicians when we returned from our trip back east.

That summer would be the final time that we would enjoy Lou's Haven, the Connolly's cottage on White Horse Beach. As had become the routine, my mother and father would spend a few days there as well, enjoying not just their grandchildren, but their counterpart grandparents, too.

The gentle summer ocean lapping up under the cottage pilings was a remarkable sedative. Michael slept well in the front bedroom upstairs while older cousin, Sean, whom he idolized, occupied the other twin bed. Barry and I, Meaghan, and my parents occupied the multiple beds in the dorm-like space adjoining the room. We were close enough to respond to any untoward occurrence but removed enough so Michael could feel some level of freedom with his older cousin.

Grampie Sullivan and Michael spent lots of time together at White Horse. They often walked the sugar-fine sand shoreline collecting interesting rocks and shells. My father's easy going demeanor and adult-like conversations had a calming effect on his grandson. Barry and I never fully disclosed the nature of Michael's seizures or his treatment to any of our parents. We felt that since we lived 3,000 miles away, we needn't worry them about situations that they could do nothing about. I think, though, that my father knew that there was more to the story than we let on.

Grandmother Mary entertained us with her usual array of tricks and treats. Most mornings, she elicited giggles galore from Meaghan and Michael by making their father egg-in-a-cup and cutting it up for her "baby." Throughout our stay, she would pull out the latest wind-up toy or gadget that had no other objective than to make people laugh at its pure silliness. And laugh we did. Sometime each day, whenever the mood struck her, she flipped a tape in a small boom box and got one and all involved in doing the chicken dance. Later in the day, NEVER before noon of course, cocktail hour was announced with Grandmother's sauntering out to the brick and beach-sand patio balancing Grandfather's rum and Tab and a couple of beers on a swinging cocktail tray. She was a joyful woman with an incredible gift for giving of herself.

Grandfather held court on the patio from dawn till dusk. Michael got the biggest kick out of Joe's wardrobe. Bargain-hunting Nana Kae and Grandmother bought him shirts at one of their favorite bargain stores. Joe paid little mind to the fact that the shirts were inscribed with someone else's name. Michael looked forward to seeing "Ed," "Roy," or "James" sitting amongst a cadre of beach folk friends on the patio each day. Michael would join them for their discussions about the Red Sox. Since we usually visited there in August, the Red Sox discussions were generally about their end-of-summer demise. Joe had an uncanny ability to tell a story, any story, in a way that would first break him up and then break up his audience. Michael thought him quite amusing and eagerly sought out his company.

Grammie Sullivan's favorite past time–sunning–was easily accomplished at White Horse. Grandmother wouldn't allow her to do any cooking, for which I'm certain she was most grateful as she isn't exactly into the culinary arts. She was often chief of the clean-up brigade, hurrying her crew along so we could all get on with the rest of the evening. She promoted and eagerly participated in the nightly card games of twenty-one. My mother enjoyed the games most when she could kid and goad Joe, and on occasion, beat him. Meaghan and

Michael took in this ritual gathering of family and beach friends until the effects of saltwater and sun took their daily toll.

Hot days tempered by cooling ocean breezes; warm evenings under star-filled skies; family…friends…fun. White Horse was a reprieve from epilepsy's realities. We would miss its part in our lives when we could no longer take refuge there.

"Reality is something you rise above." *–Liza Minelli*

Reality Bites

My dear friend and neighbor, Suzanne, is a local pediatrician. When I sought her advice regarding a pediatric neurologist for Michael, she recommended that we talk to a recent newcomer to the Children's Hospital Neurology Group in whom she had great confidence. Mark Nespeca, she told us, did his fellowship in EEGs and was very normal (for a neurologist).

At about six feet five with a head full of thick black hair and a bearded face, Dr. Nespeca was quite an imposing figure. His ability to listen, empathy toward children and their parents, and patient explanation of seizure disorders, EEG patterns, and medication effects and side effects, are only part of his extraordinary skill set. His quick establishment of a guy-to-guy rapport with our son, "Hi Connolly, how's it going?" made Michael comfortable enough to respond, "Hi Nespeca, everything's okay". He was smart, kind, and accessible. We were convinced that Michael would be in superb hands.

Dr. Nespeca explained that Michael had at least two types of seizures—tonic-clonic (formerly known as grand mal) and atypical absence, which were absence or petit mal, "blanking out" episodes with the additional complexity of involuntary physical movements such as outstretched arms during some seizure episodes. He recommended that a drug called Depakote be added to Michael's medication regimen. As with most anti-seizure medications, the Depakote dosage would be adjusted slowly upward until a therapeutic blood level was reached, and/or seizures were totally under control.

During this upward titration process, certain side effects such as increasing drowsiness were noted, but this type of side effect generally subsided over time so there was no undue concern.

A more bothersome side effect of Depakote was the occurrence of some nausea and occasional vomiting. Michael was not reacting well to this drug. On the eve of Memorial Day, Michael awakened from sleep just prior to midnight. He cried, uncharacteristically, about abdominal pain. I thought for a few hours, he probably had contracted a nasty virus and was certain his symptoms would subside momentarily. When there appeared to be no relief in sight as morning approached, I thought the episode might be medication-related.

I rocked Michael in my arms until 6:00 a.m., which I viewed as a reasonable time to try and reach the on-call neurologist. Mark Nespeca returned my call within minutes and agreed to see us in a Children's Hospital Clinic on Memorial Day at twelve noon. Six more hours!

Dr. Nespeca met us in the clinic at 12:00 sharp. After probing Michael's abdomen and reviewing the results of his blood tests, he told me Michael had pancreatitis and would need to be admitted to the hospital.

I called Barry who had taken Meaghan to our friends', the Tremblays, for a holiday picnic. Between the swallow of my sobs, we managed to arrange for Barry to spend the night at the hospital, and I would relieve him to take the day shift the following day. Barry arrived toward evening after all the admission processes had been completed. Children's supplied a comfortable chair/bed and change of linens for Dad, the nightshift caretaker.

Michael was on NPO (no food or drink by mouth) status so his pancreas could rest. He had an IV running and had been taken off all his medications. He had an occasional pain and severe bouts of diarrhea and dry heaves, but he was reasonably comfortable. Whenever any doctor or nurse asked him how he felt, his response was always the same, "Good."

I returned to the Tremblays to pick up Meaghan. It was that night that our routine for Michael's multiple hospital stays took root. Meaghan would occupy Barry's side of the bed, I would wrap her in my arms for my comfort as much as hers, and we would sleep. In the morning, we would awaken earlier than usual so I could get her squared away at a neighbor's or friend's home before she went to school, and I could relieve Barry. Then, Barry would return home and get ready for a day at work. He'd pick up Meaghan after school, ensure her homework matters were in hand, and then, they would drive to the hospital. And so it went, over and over, until hospital discharge—many times over, in the course of our lives.

Michael's stay included an ultrasound to confirm his diagnosis, but it mostly consisted of being bound to the bed and an IV pole and numerous re-watching of the kinds of movies that appeal to seven-year-olds. I believe, in those days, it was the artistic group that included Rafael, Michelangelo, Leonardo, and Donatello of the Ninja Turtles. In truth, I liked the movies, too.

The worst part of Michael's stay occurred on day three. He had managed to dislodge his IV while playing a makeshift basketball game delivered to him by his close friend and babysitter, Dawn. She also happened to be my assistant and friend as well. The nurse assigned to care for Michael approached the IV insertion as routine. So did I. Michael had been stuck with plenty of needles for blood work in the past, and his previous IV insertion was not painful to him, so he was not fearful of the procedure. The first stick was unsuccessful and a bit painful judging from the grimace on Michael's face. Another nurse was called to his bedside. The RNs conferred. A second more painful stick resulted in a crying kid. I suggested that a call be made to the anesthesia department since they did this (IV insertions on kids) all the time. Instead, the nurses called an intern or resident. I was unhappy but I didn't want to leave Michael's side or piss off his nurses. The resident or intern (I never knew) arrived. By then, Michael was crying more vigorously; the two nurses were restraining him by all but lying on top of him, and I was beside myself. I don't remember if they got the needle in then, or if it took the group four tries. All I know is that in those moments, I felt useless. I could neither comfort my son nor confront his healthcare providers to suggest that they take a less traumatic approach. I recognized then what it could feel like to be on the other side of the healthcare system: vulnerable, afraid, and submissive.

Over the years, I have had the good fortune of having family-friendly bosses. I was able to conduct most of my administrative work as a home health agency director, from Michael's bedside. Dawn faithfully delivered my work and her good humor and support daily to Michael's room. This would be the start of still another trend during Michael's hospital stays. Dawn was allowed "in." Others, even our closest friends, were asked to stay away. If at all possible, contact with them was avoided. Dawn could see the tears, hear the anguish. To have done so with others, even the families back East, might have cracked the fragile wall of control and containment we erected around us during the crisis times of our lives.

Michael's classmates sent their colorful hand-drawn cards and sentiments to the hospital. Pleasant hours were spent reading everyone's messages and admiring (or laughing at) the variety of artwork. It was clear he would be welcomed back to his first-grade classroom. He was more than anxious to resume with school.

During Michael's hospitalization, the first priority was to stabilize his pancreas. As I recall, Diamox was administered via his IV and he remained in a seizure-free state. His Phenobarbital was resumed when food and drink were slowly introduced. Toward the end of the hospital stay, a new medication to control the absence seizures, for which Depakote had been given, was prescribed by Dr. Nespeca.

We were grateful that the initial period of titrating the new drug, Celontin, upward, would be during the summer. We were comfortable that as the new school year began, Michael's medication regimen would most likely be stable. Of course, we were wrong again. We had a lot to learn—still do—about epilepsy, medication side effects, learning difficulties, teacher prejudices, and childhood peer relationships. So did Michael.

That summer, we visited White Horse Beach for the last time. A fierce winter storm had washed away most of Lou's Haven, the Connolly's cottage, so Mary Connolly, family matriarch extraordinaire, rented a nearby cottage for our annual gathering. It wasn't the same. The ravaged surroundings were eerie. Pieces of Lou's Haven in the midst of bent concrete pilings were testimony of the power of the sea. In addition, Mary didn't seem quite right. Grandfather Joe was grouchy and ended up sleeping on the couch of the crowded rental during our entire stay. The highlight of our stay was the celebration of Mary and Joe's fiftieth wedding anniversary. Mary wanted to go on a cruise to Alaska. Joe didn't. They stayed home. We celebrated by inviting a group of family and friends to a local restaurant, and Barry made arrangements to take his mother on an Alaskan cruise the following spring.

We ended that summer's trip with my family in Springfield, Massachusetts. While there, we shared my parents' small Cape-Cod-style home with my brother Gary, his wife Lynne, and their toddler son Brendan, who were visiting from Washington, D.C. Brendan was irritable due to an ear infection and Lynne was nervous, first, about bringing him to a strange doctor, then, about getting him to take his medicine. I know I totally lacked empathy regarding the situation. I must have seemed the mean, cruel aunt as I showed her how to get Brendan to swallow his antibiotic by pinching his cheeks. (I know it's precisely what she thought as she whipped him out of my seemingly uncaring arms.) The truth was, that I had lots of experience with ear infections and knew Brendan's issue was transient and that he'd emerge intact. Meanwhile, I was simply too preoccupied with Michael's increasingly frequent early morning tonic-clonic seizures that had been occurring throughout our trip. We would have to make some medication adjustments upon our return to San Diego. Hopefully, the adjustments would have his seizures under control by the start of the school year.

Second grade started out with a new teacher, the same group of friends, and the seizures not quite under control. It was a year that featured First Communion preparation, Sunday school and elementary school Christmas productions, soccer, Little League baseball, and graduation to real pitcher baseball from T-ball.

Classroom issues began to surface this year. Evening calls to our home by Michael's teacher occurred once every month or two and generally focused on his sleepiness in the classroom. He often fell asleep during reading sessions. The teacher was close to retirement and was not generally known as a patient individual. However, based upon our experience, she was most kind, considerate, and caring. She obviously tried to accommodate Michael's needs, kept us very informed, and genuinely seemed to get a charge out of Michael's dry sense of humor. Learning problems were not overwhelming at this time. Michael "got" the rudimentary math concepts and could read, though not without a struggle.

Outside the classroom, Michael's life appeared quite normal for a seven-year-old boy. When I remarked one day in the lunchroom at work that Michael wanted to be a catcher on his baseball team, one of my colleagues looked at me askance and shrieked, "With seizures, you're going to let him be catcher?"

Until that moment, I thought that with a mask, pads, chest protector, and other pieces of equipment, catcher might be the best position for Michael. It certainly seemed to me that he'd have plenty of protection! Through all the baseball years that followed, my most unnerving moments occurred when Michael stood at the plate. Walk, hit, or strikeout, I always breathed easier when an at-bat ended with Michael upright on a base or bench. Michael played the game of the boys of summer until he was fourteen.

Michael continued to play soccer as well. Michael was still savvy at playing his position and we mightily discouraged the use of "headers" to advance the ball. After a few years, his interest in this sport waned. I observed that as his medications were increased, Michael's coordination and sense of self in space diminished. I think that is what made him grow to dislike an activity that seemed, at one time, to give him great pleasure.

My memory of certain events during this time period leaves me asking myself, "How could I do it? How could I possibly do it?" Every now and then, Michael would have an early morning tonic-clonic seizure. Following the seizure, I would let Michael sleep for another hour or so, then wake him to begin his daily routine as if nothing had occurred. I didn't act this way because I minimized or ever became used to seeing a tonic-clonic seizure. Their occurrence still leaves me unraveled and on edge for days. Yet, I was determined that Michael's life should not be dictated by the seizures. I guess it was this attitude that led me to pack him off for a school day, hopeful that a seizure would not recur as we re-adjusted dosages or changed medications. I must have had some great denial mechanism click in during those days. Fortunately, for many years, Michael did not have a tonic-clonic seizure in the school setting. He would have other types, though, and would suffer stigma related to them…but that would come a little later.

Michael's new seizure types were a bit of a mystery in terms of pigeonholing to a particular form of epilepsy. It appeared he was having absence seizures (just not "there" for five to ten seconds) and some of these would be accompanied by an extension of his arms forward or upward. Other times, he would have slight little jerks of his shoulders or head. He was conscious of these and began to refer to them as "twitches."

The majority of new seizures were observed at home. In school, they either didn't occur or were not noticed, at least by teachers. The kids undoubtedly noticed something different was occurring and, in time, began to give what they saw, and Michael, a label.

Many of my worries at this time centered on the type of "what-ifs" that often kept me awake at night. What if Michael has an absence seizure in the middle of his two-line appearance as Santa in the second grade play? What if he has a brief motor jerk while a shepherd holding his staff on the stage at the St. James Nativity reenactment? What if he has a seizure in the First Communion procession? What if he blanks out and gets hit by a fly ball in right field? Well…he spoke his brief lines as Santa Claus and though not flawless, his performance was absent a seizure. He performed without a problem as a shepherd, his staff safely held in his hand and not jerking toward anyone else.

He received his First Communion just as angelically as all the other children. He may have missed a few fly balls, but he was never hit by one! He was managing to hold his own in the classroom. Though his seizures still were not fully controlled, he was managing to live a reasonably carefree life.

Meanwhile, Barry and I were learning what the term "sandwich generation" was all about. My mother-in-law, Mary, had been diagnosed with breast cancer just prior to our previous summer's visit. At that time, she was on some type of medication and didn't tell us what was going on. (We might worry.) Later that fall, she had a mastectomy performed on one of her breasts. A month later, the same procedure was performed on the other breast. She appeared to come through both surgeries well, and did not require chemotherapy or radiation. She was up and about several weeks later, driving, cooking, and caring for Joe and her sister, Kae, as usual.

In January, Mary and Kae came to California for a visit. Mary was only in the house a few minutes when she pulled me into the downstairs bathroom and lifted up her sweater to expose her scarred chest. She seemed totally at ease with the loss of her breasts, relieved her ordeal was over, and was anxious to get on with her life.

Mary was her generous and ever-entertaining self. She seemed to ratchet up the entertainment factor during that visit. Most memorable was the sight of her in a T-shirt that had front and backside illustrations of a voluptuous bikini-clad body! How she loved parading around the house in front of the children in that attire, evoking giggles and squeals of delight. Both kids always told her, "Grandmother, you are SO funny."

From my perspective, it appeared Mary had come through two major surgeries within a month of one another like a champ. She was, after all, over eighty years old. Nothing about her appeared to be out of sorts during her visit. She and Barry excitedly talked about the Alaskan cruise he had booked for them. In fact, during that visit I was far more worried about Kae, whose dementia or Alzheimer's (neither was truly diagnosed) had left her even more unable to fend for herself. Her ever-present dependence upon Mary was very evident even as she sat primly making seemingly lucid conversation. Worried, but not terribly concerned, would sum up my feelings at the time. After all, though gainfully employed for over fifty years at a Boston newspaper and independently driving around that rotary-infested city, Kae had never made a meal or paid her own bills. Those roles were assumed by others in the household. Taking all of this into consideration, she only seemed to be marginally worse at this time. Besides, Mary was a tough cookie and would be taking care of Joe and Kae's needs for many years to come.

Shortly after the ladies returned to Brookline, Massachusetts, Joe began taking over that end of the phone conversations, allowing that Mary "Mother" was "weak, not herself, tired, in bed" or other some other excuse that would cover her absence of contact. She also stopped writing, which she had previously done on a regular basis. Joe said her writing had become "too shaky." Initially, I thought Joe may have been exaggerating to convince Barry to cancel the Alaska trip. Joe really didn't care for being without his wife for any extensive period! When the description of Mary's declining condition continued for weeks, the focus of our conversations was to ensure she was seeing appropriate physicians to determine what was happening. Clearly, what was happening was not good and appeared to be progressing rapidly in a downward spiral. The Alaska cruise plans were placed on hold.

That summer, we stayed in Brookline for a few days in the Connolly household. Mary's status was shocking. She was unable to walk steadily and relied on Joe for support including their ventures up a winding staircase to the upstairs tub. I was fairly convinced they would surely tumble downward and break their elderly necks. She talked in short sentences with a gurgling, slurry quality. She often just stared straight ahead with doll eyes lacking the luster, amusement, and twinkle they used to contain. On occasion, a glimmer of Mary-past would surface, once making a wisecrack to the pompous neurologist for whom she waited over an hour. That was an enjoyable moment, and I think she relished it as much as I did. The kids handled the change well. Michael may not have recognized the full implications, but he certainly knew his funny grandmother was not there. Meaghan was caring and loving, giving her beloved grandmother manicures and pedicures as often as she could. Barry was quietly distressed.

I viewed this family constellation and care situation as similar to many of our "nightmare" home health clients in the home care agency I managed at the time: several elders unable to care for themselves, each other, or a house, intent on keeping things that way and not wanting to hire additional help. They DID accept the intermittent visits of a nurse and therapist from the Boston Visiting Nurse Association. But these services, no matter how helpful, were not even close to the household and personal care help that could adequately maintain these three in their home. Unable to change their minds, we had to accept that they would remain in an inadequate and unsafe situation. We relied upon generous visits from my ex-sister-in-law and close young friends of

Joe and Mary to hold the pieces together. They did. Remarkably, Joe, Mary, and Kae lived out the next months of their lives in Barry's childhood home, free from serious injury and enjoying what they could of one another.

Meantime, back in California, the presence of epilepsy in our lives was increasingly evident.

"Society attacks early, when the individual is helpless." —*B.F. Skinner*

Life's Not Fair

Starting at about age four, in the course of their daily lives, my children heard me say, "Life's not fair" many times. It was commonly heard as a response to their whining about not being able to watch another TV show, play outside later, or eat dessert before they finished their meal. Eventually, both of them got the concept that they couldn't always have what they wanted any time they wanted it.

I wish so much that the phrase I repeated so often could be contained to dismay over vegetables, desserts, and playtimes. In Michael's case, he would learn the phrase's more painful meaning.

The transition to third grade was marked by transitions of medication regimens. Phenobarbital seemed to have the tonic-clonic (grand mal) seizures under reasonable control. An occasional seizure during early morning sleep would be cause to increase the dose (and increase the inattention and hyperactive behaviors, too). It was, and still is, difficult to assess what behaviors may be exhibitions of seizures, side effects of medication, or normal growth and development. At each age, Barry and I would ponder "Is it the medication? Is it just a boy thing? Is he just being seven, eight, etc. etc…?"

The daytime absence seizures that were generally coupled with a sharp tonic movement of Michael's arms forward or upward were more problematic and less responsive to medication. The force of the tonic movements could cause loss of balance resulting in thrusting forward falls. Other times, the force of the seizure would quickly and stiffly propel Michael in the direction he was going. He would continue his activity without even knowing what had occurred. It was fascinating, really, to watch them sometimes. There were many times he'd be carrying a plate or glass across the kitchen and suddenly his arms would stiffen and his body would propel quickly forward. He'd usually end up at the table or the sink with utensils in hand and food in place. Celontin was effective in decreasing such episodes for a while and then, as incidents began to increase, higher doses were tried. A soon-to-retire third grade teacher who, while kind, was not a reliable observer of in-classroom seizures or medication side-effect behaviors, replaced the vigilant teacher of second grade.

During Michael's third grade year, Barry and I were forced to recognize that we were dealing with a chronic problem medically and academically. Hopes for Michael going off seizure medications any time soon were dim. The school environment was neither as tuned in nor as supportive as in prior years. Advocating for Michael became more necessary in order to ensure his educational needs were met within our highly regarded public school.

The most disturbing occurrence of the third grade year was the erosion of Michael's friendships within his peer group. Over the years, I have done a lot of thinking regarding his difficulties with classmates. I have concluded that the ostracism and bullying experienced over the years resulted, in part, because of his classroom performance. Frequently in crying jags that he doesn't even recall now, he said kids called him "stupid" or "dumb."

Happy times as a first and second grader were replaced by the unhappiness of being left out by his former buddies and fears of being made fun of or even physically harmed by old friends. A poster made for Michael by his second grade class serves as a visual reminder of how dramatically his social life changed. The poster listed Michael's favorite foods, activities, attributes, friends, and other key second-grader type interests. It hung in Michael's room for some time after second grade. It was only in recent years I rediscovered it in his closet and noted the changes he had made: The "s" in "friends" had been crossed out in pencil so that the singular word "friend" remained; "Tom and Jason" were scribbled out and only "Aaron" remained listed. Even though I already knew about the broken friendships, my heart ached for the Michael who changed his poster. He may have been unaware of some of the happenings in his life, but sadly, his meds did not dull his sense of loss.

I am an incessant worrier by nature. It is a trait passed along by both of my grandmothers and my mother as well. I am aware I have a tendency to "overdo it." So when Michael first complained of his friends picking on him, I convinced myself it was just boy/kid stuff and that it would blow over.

One night, an emotional Michael cried to me that his friends didn't "like him anymore." The next morning, I stood at the hill above the blacktop playground and watched as he walked toward his classroom. Out of nowhere, Tom appeared behind him, cuffed him around his neck and threw Michael into a bike stand. In a moment of maternal rage, I marched down the hill over to the boy who'd been a guest in our home many times. I let him know he'd be dealing with me if he ever laid a hand on Michael again. I knew I wasn't exactly rational and that Michael might be embarrassed. I just couldn't help myself. How, I wondered, could kids be so cruel? Why was my kid the one who had to struggle against a despicable condition and now had to deal with rejection by some snotty-nosed little runts?

At the time, I viewed Tom and the other kids who were giving mine a hard time as little monsters who got away with bullying primarily because of a "boys will be boys" attitude of the school's principal. When I spoke to the principal following the bike rack incident, he told me in essence "boys should learn to take care of themselves." The day after, Michael was enrolled in a karate class for the express purpose of being equipped to defend himself.

Each day, Michael was bussed to the district's other local grammar school's after-school program. There he developed a friendship with another boy, Pat, who repeatedly asked him to transfer to his school. The other district school had enclosed classrooms versus the open environment of the one Michael had attended since kindergarten, and we reasoned that Michael might be able to focus better in such a surrounding. Since we remained unhappy about the principal's and the third grade teacher's lack of sensitivity, and Michael already had friends at the other school because of the after-care program, we enrolled Michael in the other school for his fourth-grade year.

Medication-wise, during Michael's third grade year, we tried another drug called Zarontin. The outcome was a repeat of previous drug regimens: the same pattern of ratcheting up the drug in response to multiple breakthrough seizures, thereby inducing an ever-increasing cognitive haze. Midway through the year, Dr. Nespeca prescribed yet another new drug called Felbatol. While Michael never became seizure-free during his time on it, his daytime tonic episodes decreased to about two per week. At the time, the side effects were far more acceptable to us than the drugged-up state Michael was in at high doses of Celontin and Zarontin.

Each day seemed to bring a new challenge that was a stressor not only on Michael but on all of us. The previous year, I decided that we needed to begin having "real" vacations in addition to our annual trips back East to visit our extended family. Our first attempt at this new concept was a spring break vacation to Yosemite. The idea was that the Connolly family unit needed time to enjoy life away from the hassles of the education, medication, and healthcare issues that were beginning to dominate our lives. We could enjoy one another and whatever city, country, or nature site we visited. We would briefly minimize the day-to-day epilepsy-related situations. We would escape.

The Yosemite trip solidified a family commitment to continue a tradition. Each new year would mean a new vacation destination, preferably at spring break, but an occasional summer excursion beyond the obligatory family trip would also be added. As years passed, Barry and I became even more convinced that since the bulk of Michael's life consisted of pretty lousy school/learning and health issues, we needed to make a concerted effort to interject more positive experiences. It wasn't just for Michael, though. Our vacations enabled all of us to take much-needed breaks from reality. Yosemite, Sedona, Hawaii, Washington, D.C., and Ireland would provide pleasure, lasting memories, and a renewal of spirit for all.

Barry's mother died shortly after our return from Yosemite. Barry had traveled to Boston several months earlier when Mary was briefly hospitalized. At that time, her mental deterioration was such that she did not recognize him. He bid farewell to the Mary we knew and loved during that trip. We hoped she would pass away peacefully and painlessly. Several months later, she did.

Barry returned to Boston for Mary's memorial service. She, Joe, and her sisters Anne and Kae, had willed their bodies to Harvard Medical School. I was always a bit puzzled by these staunch Catholics making a decision that prevented them from having the traditional wake and rosary services and funeral masses complete with draped caskets and incense. Nonetheless, a simple church service and household gathering of family and friends would bid Mary adieu.

Again, because of the turmoil within the Connolly-Geoghegan household, Barry did not share the extent of Michael's medical problems that we were dealing with 3,000 miles away. He attended his Mom's services alone. That pattern, too, would repeat itself.

Later that spring, Barry told Joe of our intent to travel to Ireland with the kids that summer. Joe was surprised and told us he was disappointed we would not be having an extended stay in Boston. Then, he promptly scheduled himself for cataract surgery on the day of our scheduled Boston departure. My ex-sister-in-law, Mary Ellen, who lived by Joe and carefully monitored his and Kae's health states and living conditions, remarked, "Well...I wish **I** could go to Ireland." I thought I detected a little resentment, but since she clearly did not know the whole picture, I let the remark go. In the context of my family's life, I affirmed that neither she, Joe, or anyone else could make me feel guilty about putting my family first.

We flew into Hartford, Connecticut two days prior to our scheduled departure to Ireland. We attempted to get over our West to East Coast jet lag at my parents' home in Springfield. We were a little concerned because plane rides and time changes sometimes had a negative effect on Michael's epilepsy. On the date of our scheduled nighttime departure, we visited with Joe in Boston as he recuperated from his eye surgery. He got in a couple of good-natured and direct-hit digs about traveling so far when we could just "stay put", but all in all, he seemed to enjoy seeing us and the children.

Kae was deteriorating more mentally. It was apparent that Joe and she really needed the live-in assistance that Mary Ellen had secured through a local agency. It was odd to see brother and sister-in-law without the common bond who had joined them. Mary's presence in the home was still palpable. Though the house was still very much occupied, I thought it was achingly empty without her.

We arrived in Ireland on a gloriously clear day. Forty shades of green were visible from the air as we passed over farmlands approaching our landing at Shannon airport. Jet-lagged and exhausted, we showered, took short early-morning naps, and headed to the beautiful Cliffs of Moher. The next day, we traveled from our lakeside inn outside of Limerick to an out-of-the-way, aging manor estate well outside of Cork city. I discovered during that journey that my route planning for this trip was a bit off. What appeared to be a two hour jaunt on the map, turned into four and five hour drives on sometimes harrowingly narrow, curvy roads. During these lengthy road trips Michael kept us alternately amused and annoyed by speaking *only* in his version of an Irish accent. Each day, we would explore Ireland's beauty and history as we traversed the country's southwestern coast. From the enchanting thatch-roofed cottages of Adare to the wild, desolate shorelines of Dingle Peninsula, we took in the Irish people's enjoyment of life's simple pleasures. We slowed to their pace; often out of necessity as we watched from our car windows as a herd of cows passed or an errant sheep crossed from one grazing mountainside to another. Our accommodations were considered "country and coastal inns." They were quaint—the largest was thirty-eight rooms, the smallest, seventeen. All served us the full Irish breakfast of sausage, eggs, juice, assorted cereals, and the ubiquitous brown bread slathered in creamy white butter. The charming dining rooms of these small lodgings served up some of the finest food we ever had. And, they had fine wine lists as well. The cozy pubs welcomed children and ours were particularly happy to watch two World Cup soccer games surrounded by Irish men, women, and children cheering on their national team.

Our visits to castles, farms, seaside museums, and stunning mountain-to-sea vistas instilled a sense of peace and connected us to our family roots and to one another. Michael had only two daytime breakthrough seizures during the week, but Barry who bunked with him in the small twin-bedded rooms, reported very restless nights.

For us, the trip was a resounding success. We could not know how much we would need to draw from its memories of peace and wholeness in the upcoming year.

Just prior to the start of Michael's fourth grade year, I heard a radio report about a popular new epilepsy drug being called back off the market due to an unacceptable number of incidences of aplastic anemia and deaths among patients. Frantic, I called Dr. Nespeca's office. He reluctantly advised that we should take Michael off the drug until the risks were thoroughly evaluated. We agreed to withdraw the Felbatol and begin a course of Klonapin which was not the drug of choice for several reasons but had been demonstrated effective in the short-term treatment of seizures such as Michael's. It was then that our descent into hell began.

"Fall Seven Times, Stand Up Eight." —*Japanese Proverb*

The Lost Year

"Timing is everything," my friend and mentor Sonya used to say. The timing of Felbatol's recall by the FDA, really, really sucked. In order to withdraw Felbatol relatively quickly, Dr. Nespeca prescribed a drug called Klonapin as a replacement. We were rapidly running out of drug options and Michael's mixed bag of seizures did not lend itself to treatment by some of the more traditional seizure drugs. Since the time of his initial diagnosis, Michael had remained on Phenobarbital. It was the add-on drugs that always seemed to be the problem. This time...Klonapin.

Each time a new drug was prescribed, I would run to the trusted bible recommended by Dr. Nespeca, *Seizures and Epilepsy in Childhood: a Guide for Parents*, by Dr. John M. Freeman of Johns Hopkins. I may have been uncomfortable at the time that Klonapin was in the same sedating family as Valium and Ativan. I don't remember. I **do** know that by the time the first day of fourth grade arrived just after Labor Day, Michael was duller, more listless, more irritable, and less like himself. Years later, I read that Stevie Nicks credited this same drug for her eight-year lapse of songwriting creativity. Oh Stevie...if I only knew!

Michael's fourth-grade teacher was, to use a term I'm quite fond of, a "piece of work." She was a gray-haired, attractive, forty-something woman who was experiencing marital woes with her twenty-something spouse. However well intentioned she may have been, her mind was generally not on her classroom and most assuredly was not tuned in to detect seizure activity in a relatively quiet, unobtrusive student.

Michael struggled, we struggled. School was tough. The teacher used an overhead projector to display homework assignments. Michael was lucky if he got even half of the material copied. Efforts to get her typed assignment sheets were not successful. The utilization of the overhead for teaching various subjects resulted in Michael's having sparse notes and little retention of what was discussed.

Meanwhile, Michael became more "fogged up" as Klonapin doses were increased to try to control the escalating number of seizures he was experiencing. In fairness to his teacher, I will say it was very difficult during this time to differentiate an absence seizure (blanking out) from the zoned-out state created by the Klonapin. No matter what types of teaching techniques were applied, they were still directed toward a kid whose brain was simply unable to function with any degree of normalcy.

On November 4th, I received a phone call at work from the school's nurse. Prior to that time, I had come to rely upon and trust her judgment. She reported that Michael was sleeping in her office and that I should come to pick him up, as he seemed unable to complete the school day. I arrived at the school and found a snoring Michael on the cot in the nurse's office. The nurse related that the teacher told her Michael had fallen asleep in class so she carried him "dead weight" to the office. Michael was absolutely unarousable. He had no response to shouting, no response to painful stimuli. I carried him from the office and drove the three minutes to my home to call Dr. Nespeca. His responsive staff connected me to him immediately as my weekly housekeeper, Maria, was gently slapping Michael's face trying to get him to respond.

Following a brief discussion during which I bordered on hysterical, Dr. Nespeca suggested I drive to Children's Emergency Department and he would meet us there. About ten minutes later, on our drive, Michael opened his eyes and slowly spoke a few words. I phoned Dr. Nespeca from the car and he told me we should come directly to his office. Upon our arrival in the neurology suite, we were immediately ushered to a room whereupon Dr. Nespeca determined that a then mildly reactive Michael was in a state called "status epilepticus." This is a dangerous situation that warrants immediate intervention. I recognized the seriousness of the situation when April, an EEG technician who had taken a fancy to Michael over the years, began to cry when he had about four tonic seizures in quick succession. I thought then, "Damn, she's seen it all and she's coming apart." I tried to maintain a sense of calm. Michael was admitted to the hospital.

43

Michael remained mildly responsive in Dr. Nespeca's office and throughout the transfer to the hospital unit. Dr. Nespeca ordered his medications. Michael was alert enough at the time that Dr. Nespeca ordered oral medications.

I sat on Michael's bed viewing his EEG, watching his gauze-wrapped head as he began to drift off into a less coherent state. Repeatedly, I asked the assigned nurse (I'll call her "J") to get his medications. Repeatedly, she told me the meds were on their way from the pharmacy. It took three hours to deliver drugs up one flight of stairs! When the drugs finally arrived, Michael was once again in full-blown status epilepticus and I was once again feeling rather helpless and vulnerable. Should I have driven home to get his meds? Even with a half hour coming and going, I could have gotten his meds to him in a more timely manner. But that would mean leaving him in "J's" hands, not a good idea. She had, after all, already attempted to give him one medication that was not prescribed for him. Who would know what could happen if I were not there?

Michael was going to have to be rescued from this situation by the IV administration of Ativan. Small doses would be given every hour, then every two hours until he stabilized.

Michael had been placed in a two-bed room in the specialty care unit. Given my healthcare experience and the anger, agitation, and anxiety I was having over the medication delivery incident, it was clear to me this room arrangement would be unacceptable. Obviously, Barry or I would need to be present twenty-four seven. The managerial staff had no problem accommodating my single room request. Michael, Barry, Meaghan, and I would adapt as best we could to Michael's room in Children's Hospital in November of 1994.

The family quickly and smoothly shifted to the hospital routine. Barry and Meaghan arrived at dinnertime. Michael, who had "awakened" several hours after the start of Ativan, ate his hospital dinner menu items and Barry, Meaghan, and I dined on take-out from a variety of drive-throughs in the hospital area. Michael didn't mind. He was generally pretty zoned out due to seizures or Ativan. It astonished me he could respond to even simple questions in the first couple of days. But there he was giving the correct answers to simple addition and other questions various doctors would ask to ascertain his level of consciousness.

After dinner, Meaghan and I returned home. She completed the eighth grade homework that she started in the hospital, and then she would occupy Barry's side of the bed as I wrapped her snuggly in my arms taking as much comfort from her as I was hoping to give. Oddly, I could sleep through those nights.

Barry secured sheets and pillowcases from the hospital unit's linen room and prepared a special parent's chair for nighttime watch. Just as I did during the day, he would keep track of the number of Michael's tonic seizures. During the first several days of Michael's hospital stay, the seizures were so numerous we would completely fill a narrow paper towel with our recordings per shift.

In the morning, I dropped Meaghan at a neighbor's so I could relieve Barry at the hospital. He'd return home, shower, change, and go to work for the day. Following work, he'd retrieve Meaghan and start our routine all over again.

My days were spent in the hospital, monitoring both Michael and his providers and hoping for a quick resolution to his condition. Before Ativan was given IV push, the nurses were supposed to check Michael's state of arousal. Of course, they didn't do so each time, but I, the bitch mother from hell, was there to remind them. By day three or four, it was looking like Michael would be responsive to the therapy and would probably be able to be discharged within days.

One evening, Barry told me I had received a call at home from my friend Betty. By day four of Michael's hospitalization, I felt I had the strength to call my dear friend who was in the final stages of life after a courageous battle with ovarian cancer. I called her from Michael's room. The nurse who entered during the call was very concerned because I was crying and visibly upset. I assured her it was not because of Michael's situation but was due to Betty's request that I assist two other close friends in planning a San Diego memorial service. The meticulously organized Betty (she had an organizer and referred to it as her "brain" years before most of us heard of Steven Covey) was making sure her San Diego friends had the same opportunity for closure as her Seattle-area family and friends since she now resided there. I thought, "This is all too much. I simply can't take anymore." I would have to.

When Michael could be trusted to be steady on his feet—day four or five—we started walking around the hospital, inside and out. He was horribly cranky and irritable and I was horribly discouraged and upset, so for a change of pace I suggested we start singing some oldies I thought he might like. We easily spent five or six hours in the course of a few days marching back and forth in front of Children's Hospital singing Dusty Springfield's "Wishin' and Hopin'" and, of all things, Neil Sedaka's "Breaking Up is Hard to Do." A few weeks later, one of my home care employees said she saw the two of us on the sidewalk outside the hospital, but she didn't stop because she was so touched and didn't want to spoil a special moment.

Contrary to my practice of keeping visitors away, I acquiesced when Pat's mother asked if he could visit. It was a quiet time; the two boys on the hospital bed (Michael's head wrapped in gauze to steady the EEG leads) reading a *Surfer Magazine* Pat brought. The pages they focused on were most often those with bikini-clad beach chicks. My heart was full when Pat presented Michael with an autographed Tony Gwynn baseball. I thought then, this is a true friend.

The occurrence of tonic seizures gradually ceased, and on day seven, we were given the okay to return home. Michael was still very groggy from the extensive Ativan dosages. We would have to continue it at home orally while titrating it downward.

Once we were all home and the crisis was over, we informed the grandparents. This was a pattern we had adopted over the years. Get through the immediate crisis and when things are looking a little better, let the relatives know. In any case, for many years, the Connolly, Geoghegan, McCarthy, and Sullivan clans and a multitude of friends had no clue as to the seriousness of Michael's condition or the impact it had upon our lives.

So, we returned home to resume our life. Michael returned to school but still remained in a zombie-like state for a week or two. He wasn't actively seizing so we were grateful for that. He wasn't actually learning either, and we knew not what the implications of that would be.

We had our traditional, quiet, family-only Thanksgiving and continued our practice of stating what we were thankful for before digging in. Who knows why—because he had heard it in years past, because we minimized his own situation, because we were meant to take pause—Michael said he was thankful for his "family and health." Tears squelched, we toasted and ate.

My parents arrived in early December for what was now a quite extended stay. It was clear they thought Michael was different, but as always, each of them could get a rise out of Michael in wit, activity, and discussion that few others could.

Michael began to have more breakthrough seizures. Early one morning, during my parents' stay, he had a tonic-clonic seizure. Barry had already left for work. My father was in the bathroom close to Michael's room. I called, "Daddy."

He came in and saw Michael in the final stages. I am so very sorry even to his day that I called out to him. I vividly remember catching a glance of my sweet father's face reflected later in the bathroom mirror. He was clearly distressed by what he had seen.

Grammie and Grampie Sullivan were at the heart of the traditional Christmas Eve Open House celebration. Our adopted California family of diverse friends grew to love them and anticipate their arrival. My father engaged our friends in lively political discussions (he and Don Tremblay liked to egg me on by attesting their admiration of Ronald Reagan). Dad was the official clean-up guy during and after the party. My mother took care of providing food and beverages to the "older" guests, who generally were about her age but not nearly as spry. In 1994, the occasion outwardly was a happy one. Michael's symptoms, at least for the evening, were controlled, and a fun time was had by all.

I was hesitant to go on a brief Napa Valley excursion with our friends Sonya and Dick, but since the built-in babysitters were in town, Barry and I set out for Napa on December 27th. As we pulled out of the driveway, Michael, who was in his nightshirt standing in front of Grampie, had a brief tonic seizure episode where his arms extended above his head. My father quickly shut the door but, at that moment, the vacation was over for me.

We stayed at a wonderful inn in St. Helena in a room adjacent to the Healys. We had gourmet lunches and dinners and visited lovely wineries, but Michael was constantly on our minds. I had numerous conversations with my parents and Dr. Nespeca regarding increasing the Ativan dosage. I was a wreck. I was distressed I was at such a distance. I was consumed with an awareness of how much Michael's epilepsy and the failure of treatment had taken over our lives.

When we returned home, Michael had not improved. School resumed after the holiday break but Michael was not in attendance. He was having ten or more breakthrough tonic seizures a day. Dr. Nespeca said we could go into the hospital or we could opt to try and reverse the situation with increasing doses of Ativan at home. I opted for home. My dad somewhat reluctantly

47

returned to Massachusetts so he could golf in Connecticut with his buddies and my mom stayed to provide much-needed support. The day before my dad left, he and Michael were practicing on Michael's skateboard in the driveway. Michael wore a helmet and miraculously had no seizures while playing. Grampie, on the other hand, slipped off of the skateboard, bounced off the driveway with his wrist and caused my heart to race.

"Please," I said, "don't hurt yourself. I can only deal with one of you guys down at a time."

Michael remained home for a full two weeks after school re-started. I was recording the number of seizures per day and stopped when it got to twenty-six before noon one day. My mom was great. She talked calmly to Michael, watched multiple movies with him, and enabled me to make an occasional errand out of the house. Fortunately, none of the seizures were tonic-clonic so she didn't witness what my father had seen.

Michael contracted yet another sinus infection. A trip to the ENT specialist, Dr. Pransky, confirmed the diagnosis. Dr. Pransky felt that a washing out of the sinus tracts (lavage) might help not only the sinuses, but would probably reduce the occurrence of seizures, since infections generally compromised Michael's seizure threshold.

Dr. Pransky wanted to arrange the outpatient operative procedure immediately. It was a procedure that would require authorization through my insurance company. When I was told at the pediatric office that managed care approval could take up to ten days minimum, I took matters into my own hands. Seated in my living room watching Michael watch the movie *The Client* for about the seventh time, while having a tonic episode every few minutes, I dialed the insurance company's customer service number. I explained the situation and was told by the young man on the other end "appropriate procedures must be followed—the utilization review will take place in about ten days." I asked to speak with a supervisor. I was told no one was available. I asked the insurance company phone-answerer to relay a message to his supervisor with the expectation that I would receive a return phone call within ten minutes. My message indicated that the procedure requiring authorization could more easily be accomplished as part of Michael's therapy if he were an inpatient. I reminded the insurance company phone-answerer that Michael's one hundred seizures a day indeed qualified him for an inpatient stay and that I had no problem racking up another $13,000 bill (what the hospital charged in November). I left Michael with my mom to pick up Meaghan at the bus stop and when I returned, I received a message authorizing an approval for surgery the following day. What, I wondered, do the poor people without healthcare system savvy do? The alarming answer…they wait, they watch kids seize, suffer with pain, and grow weaker as they wait for approval from the paper-pushing guardians of the health plan's dollars.

Dr. Pransky greeted Barry, Michael, and me the next day in outpatient surgery. We all agreed that a little anesthesia might have calming effects on Michael's brain. The surgery went smoothly. Whether coincidental or contributory, after the surgery, Michael's seizures began rapidly decreasing in number. By the third week of January, Michael could return to school. He was neither alert nor seizure-free, but he was vastly improved.

The evening of my forty-fourth birthday, January 23, I dined out with three of my friends. Even though my family's life had been turned pretty much upside down in the prior few months, I somehow felt luckier than my meal mates who spoke of breakdowns, bankruptcy, and job losses. By birthday celebration standards, it was pretty much a bummer, but I will always remember that I left the group that evening feeling pretty lucky about my life.

At 6:45 the next morning, I could hear my mother speaking loudly into the phone. She was due to travel back to Massachusetts two days later and had called to finalize airport pick-up plans with my dad. "Mary Lou, come down here. Something's wrong with your father. Talk to him."

"Hi, Daddy. How are you?"

"Yes," he replied.

"Are you okay?"

"Yes," he replied again.

"Daddy, is anyone else there?"

"Yes," again.

"Daddy, can you say anything else?"

"Yes." Silence.

I directed my mother to stay on the phone talking to my father while I grabbed my cell phone from the car and phoned my aunt Marion. I asked Marion to cross the field that separated her home from my parents', check my father out, and get him to the hospital. I suspected he had a stroke. We kept my father on the phone until Marion and my Uncle Charlie arrived and they agreed something indeed was wrong and they'd get him to a hospital.

Things progressed quite rapidly after that. I called my dad's youngest sister, Kathleen, who is a nurse, to alert her to the situation. She would take care of things at that end until my mom and I or one of my brothers arrived.

Then, I called my boss, Mary, who was understanding and sympathetic, urging me to do whatever was necessary.

I called Barry and let him know I'd be gone when he returned from work and he'd have to pick up both kids and break the news to Meaghan.

Hurriedly, I transported Michael to school, trying to maintain my composure so he wouldn't be unduly worried. As dazed and confused as he was during those days, he does recall that morning. Before leaving the house, he gave me his good luck troll to give Grampie to help him get well.

Then I called the airlines, changed my mom's flight, and booked one for myself. Lastly, I called Dawn to take us to the airport and to continue to try and contact my brother Gary in Washington, D.C. if we weren't successful before our flight took off. Gary was the closest of my three brothers to Springfield, Massachusetts. I was desperate for one of us to get there as quickly as possible. Who knew what might happen?

I was holding myself together for my mother. I lost all composure, however, when the American Airlines ticket agent behaved so kindly toward me. God, was I fragile!

While I was on the public phone in the airport trying to reach my aunt, Dawn was still tying to locate Gary at the Capitol. His job duties as an aide on the House Administration Committee had recently changed due to the takeover of committee activities by Congressman Gingrich. Dawn was transferred multiple times to people who had no clue where my brother might be. Her exasperation was apparent to the operator who occupied the last stop on the transfer roster. My mother and I stood by her as she was asked what she (Dawn) wanted her (operator) to do. "I want you to find him, goddammit.

You *are* the fucking government," she yelled. She looked up at us, gave us a little righteous nod of her head, and we all had a tension-releasing, tear-producing belly laugh.

The cross-country trip was lengthy. Conversation was limited. Any discussion of what might be going on brought one or the other of us to the brink of tears. To try and talk of anything else was silly.

Kathleen and her husband Frank picked us up at the airport and filled us in. She related that my dad had experienced a heart attack and a stroke. He was unable to speak many words. It appeared the heart damage was mild to moderate. He was still undergoing tests. Gary had arrived from D.C. mid-afternoon and Charlie and Marion were at the hospital as well.

We entered my dad's hospital room. Other than looking a little pale and clammy, the only sign of illness was the oxygen cannula attached to his nose. We hugged his ruggedly handsome face and took our places at his bedside, relieved that it looked as though he would weather this, his first health crisis. That evening, I lay my head on his chest and he stroked his hands through my hair. It felt peaceful, calm, comforting. I believed everything would be all right.

Gerry arrived from Chicago. Brian was in court in Los Angeles on a DEA case. For a week, my mom, Gary, Gerry, and I ensured someone was always with my dad. He couldn't speak for himself, plus as a healthcare professional, my personal bias is that one should never, ever leave loved ones alone in hospital rooms. One morning I awoke to whispers and laughter coming from my father's bed. Kathleen was at his ear, "Look at her Ray…she's supposed to be keeping an eye on you and she fell asleep on the job". Kathleen and I giggled, and my father smiled broadly.

We were all upbeat. My dad looked great, was getting stronger, and was signed up for outpatient speech therapy. Apparently, a plaque clot dislodged during his heart attack and caused the cerebral injury that left him aphasic. We were feeling so optimistic we bought Superbowl T-shirts, pizza and soft drinks and watched the game in my father's hospital room as the San Francisco 49ers soundly trounced my San Diego Chargers.

Gary left town before my dad was discharged from the hospital. Gerry and I took the same plane to Chicago the day after my father returned home. My mother seemed to have the Coumadin routine and speech therapy schedule down pat. Dad looked well though he still had trouble swallowing and seemed so very vulnerable without the ability to articulate his thoughts. Dad's brother, Bob, and his wife, Helen, arrived at my parents' home to take Gerry and me to the airport. My father stood up in the den and wrapped me in a hug.

"I love you," I said.

"I love you, too," he easily replied.

I cried like a baby all the way to the airport. Bob and Helen tried to offer comforting words. I just couldn't shake a feeling of utter helplessness. Gerry and I had a somber flight to Chicago, each trying to put together a plan to get back to Springfield again soon. Once I was airborne to San Diego, the tears returned. I needed to get rid of them before I saw the kids, so they could maintain their positive outlooks that their Grampie was going to be just fine.

Both children were shaken. They had lost Barry's mom, Grandmother, not quite a year before and were still adjusting to the absence of her warmth and wit.

Late on the night of February 13th, my Aunt Kathleen called. I knew, of course, the news wasn't good. She was measuring her words and taking deep breaths on the other end. My father had another stroke. This time, he was weak on his right side, and early indicators were that this stroke was more extensive.

I flew home on the 15th and was met at the airport this time by my Aunt Peggy, my Mom's younger sister who is also a nurse. Peggy's usual upbeat personality was subdued and somber. She prepared me as best she could. I spent the next week in the company of all my brothers. We took shifts with my mom beside my semi-comatose, partially paralyzed father. When I called home, I tried to prepare the children.

"He would never want to live this way," I said.

They did not agree, of course. They had months to prepare for Grandmother's death since her condition deteriorated over the span of a year and they witnessed her debilitated status. But Grampie was another story... the last time they saw **him**, he was on a skateboard.

My father died on March 10th, 1995. The fire department honor guard, the procession to the cemetery led by a fire engine and marching firemen in their dress uniforms, and the bagpiper who signaled the start of the funeral Mass, were reminders of the loss of a dignified and special man. The Catholic rituals were oddly comforting to me, and the typically Irish celebration of life after the services was a start of the healing process. When I returned to Barry and the children in California, they shared their grief and enveloped me with love. Surely, I thought, we have had our share of sorrow and strife for the year.

Michael's breakthrough seizures started to increase in intensity and frequency after my return. In April, my concern grew and I attempted to contact Dr. Nespeca. This time, he was not the neurologist on-call and his colleague suggested I visit Michael's pediatrician. Dr. Eastman was always clear about her limitations in treating Michael's seizures. Her colleague, Dr. Rubenstein, who was covering for her when we showed up at the office, was quite convinced he too could not handle them after he watched five tonic episodes occur in the space of minutes. He flew out of the exam room and demanded (we could hear him) that the neurology office see us immediately.

Michael and I were whisked out of the neurology waiting room into an exam room upon our arrival fifteen minutes later. Dr. Schultz took about two minutes to determine an immediate hospital admission was warranted. Michael again was in status epilepticus. I asked if Michael could be placed on a different hospital unit. I had written a rather scathing letter after the last hospitalization and was quite certain it was now part of Michael's medical record. I wanted no repercussions, no additional problems.

Michael was admitted to a different patient-care unit. Dr. Nespeca took over the neurology oversight. Even Dr. Pransky stopped by to deliver his opinion regarding sinus issues and their possible role in creating the problem. A very insightful nurse suggested that I supply the admission history information to her, the resident, and the intern assigned to Michael at the same time. She recognized I was clearly close to breaking and had the smarts and compassion to save me from painful retellings.

This hospital stay lasted a week. During his stay, Michael was started on a newly released drug, Lamictal. It appeared to be the answer to seizure control at the time.

Michael would complete his fourth-grade year having missed seven weeks of classes due to the hospitalizations and home treatment for status epilepticus.

There is no accounting of the days missed due to over-medication and seizures. Nevertheless, the teacher's recommendation that he not proceed to grade five surprised us since we were conscientious about his keeping up with assignments and she had never broached the subject with us. Following a meeting with the school's principal and the district psychologist, it was determined Michael could attend a local private school's summer session to catch up in math and he would undergo testing to determine an individualized education plan (IEP) for his fifth grade year.

Another summer—another summer school. More than school would be visited upon us during the summer of 1995. The year from hell was only half over after all.

Early in the summer of 1995, Joe Connolly was diagnosed with an abdominal aneurysm. He called to ask for my advice since the surgeon had given him options. The first option was not to treat the aneurysm. The surgeon told Joe he could live months, even a year, before it might rupture. He also told him that death from the aneurysm burst would likely be instantaneous. The second option Joe was considering was surgery. Due to the nature of the aneurysm, the potential complications were numerous. I measured my words carefully, advising the non-treatment option. Joe listened and later, scheduled his surgery.

This time, it would be Barry who traveled eastward several times. First, to be with his father for the initial surgery and what appeared to be a routine recovery and recuperation, then to re-visit during Joe's lengthy, complication-ridden hospital stay, and finally, to be with Joe as he lay dying, and then, mourn his loss.

Out of Sync

During Michael's fifth-grade year, Meaghan was adjusting to high school. She was delighted to be out of junior high, and according to all accounts, the transition was smooth. Her biggest disappointment was not being selected for the highly competitive freshman soccer team. My maternal haunches up, I could not fathom how the coach could overlook such a smart position player. While not the fastest or fiercest, in my mind, she would have been an asset to any team. In a strange way, she derived the greatest comfort from my remarks about the coach's obvious lack of intelligence. Aside from my verbal tirades that I knew cheered her up, I was a little worried that Meaghan's self-esteem was dealt a bit of a blow. I conscientiously made an effort to ensure this one rejection would not define her sense of self. I had one child suffering blow after blow to his self-esteem. I didn't want another.

While Meaghan continued to surround herself with the same group of friends with whom she started kindergarten, Michael was again adjusting to life on the outside of the "in" group. The social ostracism would be the toughest part of the next two years. It was extremely challenging for me to meet the various soccer moms whose sons now shunned mine rather than befriended him. I wanted to ask the moms if they realized Michael was suddenly no longer a part of their sons' lives. I wanted to ask them if they knew how much their sons' actions could hurt someone. I wanted to shake each and every one of them till their perfect blonde heads were a disheveled heap. Instead, I made small talk. If asked, I'd reply Michael was "fine." Most times, I wasn't asked.

Academically, things weren't bad considering the lack of foundation of the fourth grade. An after-school tutor, who was a former schoolteacher, was secured for twice weekly sessions. She tutored Michael in math, English, and occasionally, in history. As most adults who get to know him do, she became very attached to Michael and enjoyed working with him. In the classroom, he worked with an astute special education instructor during the math session. He was one of several students who worked with her so he was less inclined to feel singled out.

Lamictal gave us a reprieve from daytime breakthrough seizures. Many times, we would go weeks, even months, without having to adjust the dosage. Nighttime seizures remained—often occurring several times during the night. Surely, the combination of two drugs with increasing dosages, coupled with restless and disturbed sleep, was not a good thing. But, for a change, we were blessedly without worrisome daytime seizures, and however groggy at times, Michael was more alert and aware than in the previous year. Another example, I guess, of what becomes acceptable when dealing with a chronic and, at times, a debilitating condition.

Every now and then, Michael would exhibit an unacceptable behavioral pattern. He became more argumentative at home especially toward his sister but sometimes toward Barry or me. Minor disagreements about homework could escalate to near rages where it was next to impossible to carry on a reasonable conversation. Frayed nerves and spirits followed these episodes. Was it medication? Should we be getting him off Phenobarbital? Was he just "letting it (rage) out" as my friend Suzanne suggested? After all, my doctor friend counseled me; "He has a lot of things to be mad about." I usually threatened counseling after such incidents but I was pretty half-hearted about it. I felt we'd overcome this obstacle, too. Besides…this wasn't routine behavior, it was the exception to the routine. But other behaviors, particularly those of an impulsive slant began to appear. A couple of these incidents were provoked by anger and annoyance. Yet, in each case, we dismissed them as boyish acting out. In retrospect, perhaps we should have moved sooner to assess what was going on with Michael. In one case, though, however immature, we experienced a feeling of sweet revenge.

The first incident involved Michael's former friend Pat, and occurred during the fifth-grade year. One night, Michael seemed to be favoring the fingers of his right hand. When pressed for an explanation at the dinner table, he explained he had jammed his thumb on his basketball while shooting hoops earlier in the evening. Suzanne, visiting at the time, examined Michael's hand and pronounced she thought he had a "boxer's fracture." An X-ray the next day confirmed her diagnosis. Michael wore a cast for three weeks. Following the casting procedure, he fessed up to his father that he hurt his hand while landing a punch on Pat. As Barry quietly told me later that evening at the kitchen counter, we could not quite repress the "Good enough" and "Go Michael" that came out of our respective mouths. Not being totally irresponsible, however, we admonished our son and tried to impress upon him that life's problems are not solved by physical violence. We hoped that his karate classes would assist him to develop better control of his emotions.

Flash forward to the sixth grade which was marked by acceptable classroom performance buoyed by in-classroom assistance and after-school tutoring, a few classmate friendships, continuing ostracism by the boys he WANTED to be friends with, acceptance by the peers on his baseball team, the reliable neighborhood friendships of Adam and Trevor, and increasing dosages of Phenobarbital and Lamictal. Michael just wanted to get through the year. So did we. We almost made it till year's end without incident.

The Friday before Mother's Day, Meaghan called me at work to report a phone message. An incensed mother had called and told Meaghan that Michael cut off her daughter's pigtail. I told a few people at work and they howled with laughter. They all knew and loved Michael and viewed this as Michael "being a boy." After speaking with the girl's mom, and assuring her that Michael would be strictly dealt with, I set out to justly punish him. I grounded him for the weekend including our annual family Mother's Day celebration at the San Diego Padres baseball game.

"This will teach him," I thought.

I took Meaghan and two of her girlfriends to the game but I quickly learned that a Mother's Day without half the family is pretty hollow and not a lot of fun. Michael seemed appropriately penitent and by the end of the weekend, we were fairly confident a lesson had been learned.

Several weeks later, I volunteered in the makeup room at Michael's sixth-grade play. There, I met the girl who so annoyed my son he had cut off a portion of her pigtail. I say "portion" because I had the opportunity to fully examine her blonde locks as I prepared her hair for the stage and I could not tell there was any hair missing. As the young actress made her way jumping around the room in and out of everyone's face, I understood how she could cause some annoyance though I was sure not to share such thoughts with my son.

Finally, graduation day arrived. My heart ached as I watched Michael still try to continue to interact with the boys who clearly did not want him around. I hurried us out of the gathering and treated him to a special lunch and a movie. Maybe the drug-induced fog is a good thing, I thought. Maybe it dulls the rejection pangs. Maybe he doesn't notice at all. That was surely wistful, wishful thinking on my part.

That summer, adding insult to injury, one evening our home was toilet-papered. I groaned as I backed the car out of the driveway. Somehow, I knew this was not a good-natured neighborhood prank. Later that morning, a call from Meaghan to my workplace confirmed my suspicions. While she was in the front yard picking the place up, the culprits (former friend Pat and his friend James) walked by laughing and talking about what they'd done. They saw Meaghan too late. After she called, I really pondered what to do. Would any cause be served by confronting this? These kids ostracized and humiliated Michael for two plus years. Wasn't that enough? What kind of kids were they? I decided to call their moms. James's mother was outraged, first, because of his behavior, secondly, because her son snuck out of the home he was sleeping over to do this and she couldn't understand how that could be. Pat's mom delivered a handwritten note of apology. James arrived in person that evening with his mom at his side and he apologized. Michael never knew about the incident or the apologies. True, it was a childish prank, but it was the mean-spirited intent that really bothered me.

I think back on these incidents and chuckle about some of the circumstances now that impulsive acts and anger episodes are firmly behind us. I may second guess occasionally about when we decisively handled Michael's outbursts, but I never second guess my outrage and disturbance regarding the hurt that can be inflicted by children upon children, with words and deeds. Indeed, kids can be cruel.

"Character—the willingness to accept responsibility for one's own life—is the source from which self-respect springs." *—Joan Didion*

One Step Forward, Two Steps Back

The springtime of Michael's sixth-grade year was intense with the search for a middle school to give him a good foundation for high school. We knew the local junior high was out. Our bright, independent daughter couldn't stand it there. Meaghan's thoughts regarding that part of her schooling were that there were too many students and too few really involved teachers. Given his sister's reservations, we were pretty certain this was not a suitable school for Michael.

Through some acquaintances, I learned about a very small private school located in a country area east of our Del Mar home. Transcripts were sent, Michael was interviewed, and Barry and I visited and interviewed the owner of the school. We were impressed that many teachers were former engineers, scientists, and professionals from other occupations who had a desire to teach. We also were intrigued by the Mastery Learning technique they applied in mathematics…no movement to the next step until the current step is mastered. They accepted Michael. We felt we could relax about this decision. Michael could attend their summer school session and get accustomed to the layout and some of the teachers.

Prior to the end of sixth grade year, we discussed weaning Michael's Phenobarbital with Dr. Nespeca. If we did it gradually over the summer, when the year started at his new school, he would only be on one drug. We knew there were risks to withdrawal but we were willing to take them. It has long been recognized that Phenobarbital causes hyperactivity, maybe impulsivity, and we felt it may have been the root of some of Michael's occasional undesirable behaviors.

The weaning process went well for many weeks. We delighted in observing that Michael was far more alert, cheerful, and engaged.

By late July, we had nearly completed the weaning process. I traveled east with the kids while Barry remained at his job during budget season. I noted early during the first week of our stay at my mom's when Michael and I were in adjoining rooms, that he was having an increase in brief, nocturnal, tonic seizures—often six to ten per night. Later in the week, my mom, Meaghan, Michael, and I traveled to my Aunt Ellen's and Uncle Sam's home on Cape Cod. Michael slept in the sofa bed and I occupied the couch in an upstairs guestroom. During the night, Michael sat up with his arms extended having brief tonic seizures at least hourly. As dawn approached, one of these episodes advanced to a full-blown tonic-clonic seizure with eyes rolling back in his head, jaw clenching, mouth frothing, and limbs in spasms. After a couple of minutes, there was stillness. I was devastated. What to do now? I called Dr. Nespeca's office. He instructed me to give Michael a "loading dose" of Phenobarbital—huge dose to get started—then place him back on the dosage he was on before we began this unsuccessful weaning process.

Once again, I was shaken. It had been some time since I'd seen Michael in the throes of a tonic-clonic seizure. It is a sight not easily forgotten. Michael slept off the initial Phenobarbital loading dose and by late afternoon, joined us all for a trip to the beach and later, to a great Cape Cod ice cream stand. I minimized the seizure episode itself since I felt little would be gained by doing otherwise. Ellen's daughter Mary Ellen, a nurse, was the lone person other than Meaghan who recognized that a significant setback had just occurred.

Following the seizure episode on Cape Cod, daytime breakthrough seizures began to recur with regularity. With a new school year in a new school setting looming ahead, we were anxious to bring the obvious daytime seizures under control. Fears of what had happened in the past when two breakthrough seizures a day escalated to twenty, and then to status epilepticus, made us faithful reporters of breakthrough instances to Dr. Nespeca. Remembrance of past events also made us unquestioning followers of ratcheting up the dosages of Lamictal and Phenobarbital as prescribed by Dr. Nespeca. What else could we do? By the first week of school, Michael was dazed and confused and still experiencing breakthrough tonic seizures in which his arms suddenly flew upward or forward and loss of balance often occurred.

I picked Michael up from his new school on the Friday of his first week. I watched from my car as he had one tonic seizure on his walk across the field. Shortly thereafter, on the ride home from school, he had several more. We went immediately to Dr. Eastman's office wherein he had several more in her presence in the space of a few minutes. She advised an immediate visit to Dr. Neopeen. Before she left the exam room to make arrangements, she glanced at me, walked across the small room, and gave me a gentle hug. That is when my barrier of self-containment broke. Kindness in a word or touch could be devastating to what I viewed as a vital element of self-control.

Michael ended up in the hospital yet again. We were all too familiar with the routine: goop his head up to attach the electrodes for the EEG, wrap his head in gauze, admit him to a private room so Dad could bunk in. Then, try another method to bring him out of status epilepticus. I believe this time the regimen included the use of IV Decadron and a stab at using IVIG. One infusion was tried because of the theory that maybe there was some swelling of Michael's brain, the other, on the chance the episode might somehow be brought on by an autoimmune process. Dr. Pransky, ENT, even paid a hospital room visit to check if Michael's ears or sinuses had anything to do with this episode. In addition, once the status episode was satisfactorily resolved, Michael was placed on a new anti-seizure medication called Topamax. (I'd heard it referred to as dope-a-max by some unhappy parents.) Our primary concern at the time was to decrease Michael's seizures. By the end of a week, Michael was having one or two brief tonic seizures a day and was clear enough to follow directions and engage, though dully, in conversation. He was easily distracted, cranky, and anxious to get out of the hospital. So, we took him home with plans to increase Topamax gradually and monitor its effect upon seizure control.

Michael returned to his school in the third week of the semester, more dazed, confused, and drugged than when he arrived for his first day several weeks earlier. He was now on three heavy-duty anti-seizure medications and although he was upright and mobile, he could hardly be called fully functional. We maintained hope, though, that with the excellent teacher-to-student ratio, he could continue to learn and even succeed at school. Academically, the school was precisely what Michael needed and he performed quite well considering his medicated state. Socially, he did not connect with the students in his grade level but was friendly with several of the high schoolers including a girl named Holly who took Michael under her wing and was a kind presence on campus. Additionally, he had several excellent instructors, among them a teacher named Deborah who actually engaged Michael in the process of learning English and math. Michael played on the tiny school's flag football team, and though to outward appearances, he SEEMED to be a part of the campus activities, he frequently expressed his intense dislike of the school and insisted that when the time came, he wanted to attend a larger high school elsewhere. On that note, we could hardly disagree since the high school classes in this country-day setting usually whittled down to about six students at graduation.

Eighth grade was more of the same, and Barry and I got serious regarding the planning and decision-making process of where high school should occur. We had Michael tested by an educational psychologist during this time to ensure that wherever he wound up, he would have an education plan to meet his special needs. Through the psychologist, we were referred to Madeline Falcone who operates an educational program called the Falcone Institute where students "learn how to learn". We didn't realize at the time, the valuable role Madeline would play in our lives.

A class trip to Washington, D.C., Pennsylvania, and New York City found Barry in the role of chaperone since Michael's seizures were still a nightly occurrence and he simply couldn't go unmonitored. Barry loved the historical aspects of the trip but easily could have done without the assignment of keeping some of Michael's more unruly male classmates in line.

Graduation from eighth grade was a low-key affair with the aforementioned teacher Deborah saying special words about each graduate. Her words regarding Michael brought tears to my eyes. She was so supportive, noting he would succeed at "anything he tried…" if he just "believed in himself." Michael missed the after-grad splash in a classmate's pool because he said he didn't feel well. I suspected he didn't feel "welcomed" and thus we closed that education chapter quietly grateful for the real learning that had occurred, and saddened by the continuing lack of Michael making any real connections with his peers in the school setting.

"Drop the questions what tomorrow may bring, and count as profit every day that fate allows you." —*Horace*

Stolen Slumber

Lying in the dark, listening to the silence, it's sometimes impossible to push the bad thoughts away. Day-to-day worries are replaced by anxiety that is caused by envisioning a series of unthinkable scenarios. In the stillness, I tense up, toss my body about, and shake my head trying to free myself from images of a seizure in the shower, a lengthy tonic-clonic seizure we do not hear at night, a fall down the stairs. Then...deep breaths as I try to imagine waves lapping onto the seashore, saying over and over to quiet my racing mind, "Be still, be still, be still."

A *People Magazine* caption in the late nineties announced that the ten-year-old son of a Colorado sports figure died of an epileptic seizure. Above the brief announcement there was a picture of a smiling, adorable boy with his dad. A newspaper sports article reported about a promising soon-to-be NFL football player who fell during an epileptic seizure in the bathroom of his coach's home and died as a result of injuries incurred. A notice in Michael's high school told of the unexpected death of a teacher's younger brother. I am told upon inquiry that it is believed that the young man with epilepsy had a seizure while showering. A colleague's daughter died at age twenty-three of an epileptic seizure during sleep. An Olympic athlete stunned the sports world with her seizure-related death. A couple joined the Epilepsy Foundation Board in November of 2001. When they introduced themselves, they explained that their nineteen-year-old son had been discovered dead in his college dorm room six months earlier. He had been diagnosed with epilepsy fifteen months before. They had joined the board determined to "make sense" out of their personal tragedy. Another board member, a physician, lost his beloved wife to sudden unexpected death from epilepsy, in 2003. If such occurrences of death related to seizures are so rare, why do I know of so many in my relatively small circle of life? It is the knowledge of such tragedies and the realization that we are powerless to prevent them, that leads to the agonizing and dreadful thoughts which steal sleep as they invade and overcome my charged nighttime mind.

I hear a rustling of sheets. What's going on? I should check. I walk down the hall and peek in Michael's room. He's still. I make my way back to bed next to Barry, trying not to disturb his sleep as I restlessly tuck in again. I chide myself of course. This is what I used to do when the kids were babies...tiptoe into their rooms to assure myself they were breathing.

Later, I hear a groan. Was that a movement? This time I pick up my pace down the hall. Michael's breathing is heavy now. He's noisily snoring. He must have had a brief tonic seizure. Satisfied it's over, I retrace my steps and attempt to quietly re-enter my own bed.

As morning approaches, I hear a familiar and unwelcome sound that I liken to an old man crying out in agony. It must be 4:00 or 5:00 a.m. Barry joins me in the hallway run for these; the more lengthy and severe tonic seizures. Sometimes, they last a minute or two and sometimes longer. We can go back to our bed after the five to fifteen second tonic seizures now. We can even manage to close our eyes–sleep after them–most times. But the aftermath of the longer-lasting tonic seizures is a different story. First, there is the pure visceral fear of seeing your child's body writhing, eyes rolling back, lips turning blue. When will he take a breath? How long will this last? How long is TOO long? We watch...count...cradle him in our arms. Then there is the relief; it's over. But it's not really over. His body is exhausted, the mind spent. Sleep, baby, sleep. I will stay by you till your heart stops racing and you are peaceful in your post-seizure state.

How many seizures are too many in a night? What does this do to the brain? How will they impact Michael's function tomorrow, next week, next year? Will there ever be a treatment these seizures respond to? What if we don't hear a seizure? What if we're not here? What if they never become controlled? What if...

Oh, yes, nighttime...in addition to the chronic worry and anxiety, it's also the perfect environ for second guessing. Barry has said many times we shouldn't second guess our decisions. After all, they're over and done and we cannot reverse course. He does well with this mode of action. However, my nature as a "bogtrotter" (Barry's description of my pessimist side) will not allow me to peacefully accept our past choices. Thus, I lay there and fret over school choices, medication regimens, the timing of the diet, the surgery, the decision to take a year off after high school, and so on and on and on.

And, in the silence of the night, I grieve. I grieve Michael's losses: friendships and moments, days, weeks, even months of childhood and adolescence because he can't remember them. I grieve because he is not experiencing the joys of gaining independence—the ability to drive, to go away to college, to experience a first love. All that so far has been denied him, missed.

Then, finally, on some nights, sleep comes—and the spirit is refreshed to awaken to the daytime world, whatever it may bring.

"What matters today is not the difference between those who believe and those who do not believe, but between those who care and those who don't."
—*Abbe Pire*

Low School

I was driving to the Epilepsy Foundation's office the other day when I realized I had taken a different route. The route I was wrongly on happened to be the one I'd take when dropping Michael at the school he attended in ninth and tenth grades. As soon as I realized I was approaching that familiar exit, I became sick to my stomach. I suppose I could very well say I had a "gut reaction" and that pretty much sums up my feelings regarding those two years.

Of all the second guessing I have done about schools, medication changes, and alternative treatments, the decision to place Michael in an all-boy religious-affiliated school over the coed one recommended by his counselor, Madeline, is the decision I have questioned the most. It wasn't that the place was terrible or even harmful to him. It's just that it was...indifferent. Barry and I should have known better. We were simply so blown away by the recommendation of one of my work acquaintances that we failed to consider that Michael lived a thirty-minute commute away, he wouldn't know any of the boys from the religious feeder schools, he wasn't a son, cousin, brother, or nephew of an alum, and he wasn't exactly at ease making new friends.

Nevertheless, the decision was made and for one brief semester, it appeared to be a sound one. But we would learn fairly quickly that if one was not a sports jock in this school where every teacher responded to being called "coach", then one better be an all-star academician. Michael, unfortunately, was neither.

During the second semester of freshman year, the burden of a religion course in addition to the standard required curriculum, began to take its toll. Socializing at ball games, dances, and other events was out of the question since homework consumed Michael's waking hours seven days a week. Michael's individualized education plan painstakingly created by Madeline and presented to the school's academic vice principal (a little slip of a guy who habitually would not return phone calls) was virtually ignored by most teachers. Our disappointment was palpable. We had expected so much more after the parent orientation promises of a shepherd program to keep academically challenged students on track. The program was managed by a big, sweet bear of a man who was up against the odds of a culture which valued typical male behaviors, not nurturing and caring.

I viewed the culture up close and personal every Friday morning that I volunteered in the vice principal of discipline's (not his real title of course) office. Each Friday as I marched across the campus and entered the dank, musky hallways, I felt I was slicing through a thick testosterone haze. Encountering teachers was a breeze. I only had to remember to call each and every one "coach" as they stammered through small talk with the volunteer mother. IF I was fortunate enough to run into one of Michael's teachers during my campus moments, I took the opportunity to get feedback about how he was doing. The teachers, much like their academic vice principal, seemed quite averse to communicating in any way other than a catch-me-if-you-can style.

Michael completed freshman year with a high C average. We were not displeased. He attended summer school in an attempt to improve the D he received in algebra and managed to raise it ever so slightly to a low C. It seemed hardly worth the extra effort, and was a harbinger of what was coming sophomore year.

Sophomore year brought the bad S's: Spanish and Speech. No amount of tutoring could clear the conceptual fog of a foreign language and no heart rhythm relaxation techniques or kinesiology exercises could slow Michael's racing heart during speech presentations. The critique of classmates following each presentation led Michael further into an abyss of fear and anxiety. He totally missed one speaking assignment and in hopes of making up some of his lost points, read one of the readings at mandatory Friday morning Mass. I could, that morning, really feel his pain from afar. One of the worst moments of the year came when his speech teacher sent Michael to the school's counselor because he "appeared to be on drugs." WHAT? Duh, he

IS on drugs! As I spoke to the counselor the next morning in the school's courtyard, tears of anger, frustration, and hopelessness streamed down my face. Another defining moment: Michael was not in the right place.

Michael stayed and struggled to complete his sophomore year, but not without incident. One day during Spanish class, Michael's teacher prodded him for an answer. When Michael perceived that his teacher ridiculed him in front of his classmates, he ceremoniously lifted his middle finger in response and was quite unceremoniously ushered to the vice principal of discipline's office. Michael told us about it that evening before he went to his room to write an apology; a very light sentence for such an offense, I thought. However, I did chuckle silently at the apology note which said quite simply, "Dear —, I'm sorry I flipped you off." Later that week when I showed up to do my Friday morning volunteer stint, I learned Michael was regarded as something of a campus hero as he had done what many others apparently wanted to do.

The revered principal of the school succumbed to a major heart attack during Michael's sophomore year. I had truly tried during my campus times and evening school events to objectively decipher why he was so beloved. I felt only aloofness and distraction in our brief interactions. I never DID figure it out, but his packed memorial service and the overwhelming number of wet-eyed young and old men in attendance, told me I either hadn't tried hard enough or that I was one of few that the departed man had not captivated. At any rate, by year's end, Barry, Michael, and I had a discussion about not returning for junior year. Michael was adamantly opposed to changing schools again.

He said, "I want to finish where I started."

Madeline was firm in her desire to have Michael change schools. She had received little or no cooperation from Michael's teachers over the previous two years. And she, like Barry and I, felt that returning would not be in Michael's best interest. Michael gradually warmed to the idea of moving to a larger, private coed school. It too, was religiously affiliated, so would require Michael to take an additional subject. Once the decision was finalized, we were all comfortable with it, most importantly, Michael.

The replacement principal of what I glumly referred to as Testosterone H.S. had been a highly regarded college educator before his new assignment. I made an appointment to meet with him the final week of school. Better then, I reasoned, since I didn't want Michael to be the recipient of any repercussions as he finished his sophomore year. Judging from the accolades I had heard,

I thought he might want to hear an assessment of his new post by someone who had expectations going in, that remained unfulfilled on the way out. I was definitely impressed by the principal's kind and gentle demeanor and his engaging and involved conversation style. I actually felt he was listening and seemed genuinely concerned when I brought up my issues. The kindly man asked if Michael might consider returning if he promised to make things different. I actually hesitated in my response. This man MIGHT be able to change things. Then, I reminded myself of all the organizational culture classes I had taken as well as several work examples I had lived through. Reason prevailed. I recognized that changing an organization's culture could take many years and that the new principal had a formidable task ahead.

As I said before, the two years weren't the worst ever (though as I write this my stomach is experiencing the familiar butterflies). The experience probably made Michael stronger thanks to the often stinging critiques of teachers and classmates. He certainly felt cared about at least by the burley shepherd and several teachers and staff members. He did prove that he could navigate high school courses and move on to the next semester/year though it took consistent and life-consuming efforts to get a passing grade. No, it definitely was not a totally bad experience. But it was unpleasant enough to leave behind without regret.

"My dog and cat have taught me a great lesson in life...shed a lot." —*Susan Carlson*

The Arrival of Sparky

Michael had a successful first semester in high school. I had promised him, unknown to Barry, that I would get him a dog if he attained a 3.0 GPA. Well 3.0 it was, even though the A in physical ed provided balance for the D in algebra. Nonetheless, it was quite an accomplishment, and I felt Michael certainly deserved to have a pooch.

Barry was going to be a problem. "No," he said—again and again and again. Pleading and whining seemed to have no effect. He'd just repeat, "I am not going to be stuck taking care of a dog when you guys quit on the job." Well, THAT was insulting.

Undeterred, I silently searched the Internet rescue sites. At least I could tell myself that this part of my quest was well intentioned. Why get a puppy when so many unwanted creatures were waiting for a loving home? I settled on a lab since I was fairly averse to the small-dog types that Barry referred to as "rats on leashes." Yep, we would have a "real" dog!

I admit I was sneaky and not being fair to Barry when I started showing Michael and him various pictures of labs and their personal histories as posted on the Southern Californian Labrador Retriever Rescue website. No...it just wasn't fair at all to read about poor Bear who had a hair and skin problem making him most unattractive or Molly and Shannon the beautiful, elderly lab sisters whose arthritis prevented them from going to a two-story house family. Michael focused his attention on a chocolate lab called Hank. His weight of eighty pounds was a bit frightening to me but I had to admit he was a handsome specimen. Barry knew he was beat…the campaign pressed on.

The next step in the process was to complete an adoption application. Then, a home screening meeting was scheduled with a local volunteer. "Don't," I told Barry, "even think of saying you don't want a dog."

Maria, the volunteer, arrived on time and conducted her screening interview on the patio with Barry, Michael, and me. She mentioned that she had a dog named Hansi in the car. Hansi was in transit from one foster home to another. The name rang a bell with me. I remembered Hansi was a yellow lab I had circled on the fact sheet off the Internet.

"Can we meet him?" I asked. Soon after, Hansi was fertilizing our back lawn and lying next to Michael "bonding." The interview ended. Hansi and Maria walked through the house to the front door where Hansi promptly climbed up on our white leather living room couch. A quick look let me know Barry hadn't seen. No…he was in the backyard scooping the poop.

After Hansi and Maria left, I was in quite the state. It seemed as if Hansi would be perfect. A smaller lab, he seemed quite gentle and very much at ease around Michael. Michael liked him though he professed to "hating" his name. I wondered out loud if the Rescue Association would allow us to adopt Hansi but keep him in the foster home until we returned from a spring trip we were taking to Hawaii later in the month.

Barry said, "Just call and get him if you can."

Wow! Minutes later, the deal was sealed and the Rescue League made an exception to leave Hansi in one home for several weeks. I spoke with the foster family and arranged a pick-up date upon our return from vacation.

The big day arrived, April 27, 2000. I spoke with Hansi's foster father who informed me that Hansi now answered to the name "Sparky." (Paperwork accompanying our new dog listed previous names of Oscar, Hansi, and Sparky.) I should have guessed *then,* that he might have a couple of issues. But, on April 27, Michael and I would not be deterred by any negative thoughts. There we were in Coronado picking up our new best friend, leaving behind his sobbing foster mom who declared, "He loves women." Oscar, Hansi, Sparky responded best to Sparky on the drive back to Del Mar, and he settled his head comfortably on Michael's lap in the back seat.

"This is really going to work," I thought.

Neighbors and friends were most amused by our new acquisition. Suzanne could not help laughing out loud as she heard us call his name and he lazily looked up from foot level before nodding off—again. We easily settled into a routine. I got the early a.m. walks, Michael the afternoon ones and pooper-scooper duty. I was bound and determined to prove Barry wrong. Michael and I could and <u>would</u> care for "our" dog so that Barry wouldn't be able to say that Sparky was just another thing "he had to take care of."

"I'll show him to be so condescending," I thought. At least that was the plan.

The first few nights were a bit of a challenge. When bedtime arrived, I would usher Sparky to Michael's room, then settle in my own bed down the hall. Minutes would pass and there he'd be, standing beside me breathing doggie breath in my face. I'd get up, bring him back to Michael's, close the door, and return to my room. Again, minutes later, he'd be by my side over and over and over throughout the night. I was bound and determined to break his primary attachment to me. So, over the course of several nights, Sparky and I wore a trail on the hallway carpet. Then, I caved. I already logged too many sleepless hours thanks to seizure worries. I couldn't justify nighttime ramblings for a dog. Thereafter, Sparky bedded down just underfoot on my side of the bed every night, and woke me every morning by laying his chin beside my head and gazing at me through his big, sad brown eyes.

Initially, we left Sparky in the back yard while we worked and went to school during the day. Our neighbor Kevin said Sparky barked a lot (all day) so I purchased a high-frequency noise collar to discourage him. He was cured of incessant barking within a week, though clearly his underlying needs were not resolved, as we would soon discover.

About a month after Sparky joined the household, I called Barry on my cell on the way home from work. "What do you want me to get for dinner?" I chirpily asked.

"I don't care," came the chilly reply.

"What's wrong?" I asked nervously, immediately thinking something was going on with Michael.

"Sparky was very naughty."

Careful not to chuckle at Barry's use of the old-fashioned word, I inquired about Sparky's problem. Barry related that Sparky had clawed the exterior of our patio French door. I skipped the supermarket stop and drove directly home. I honestly didn't believe my mellow yellow lab could have caused much damage, so when I tiptoed skeptically past Barry and saw the six-by-two-inch diameter gouge that went one inch deep in spots, I was astonished. I fastened Sparky's leash on and announced we were off to the vet's for a check to ensure his green-tinged teeth and paws were not damaged and to ask for a behavior consult.

The vet, Dr. Bear (really!), said it looked very much like Sparky had separation anxiety. He went on to tell me that sadly, this was a primary reason many dogs were put down due to their destructive anxiety-driven behaviors. Dr. Bear laid out four options to help:

1) doggie run with gated barriers
2) doggie tranquilizer
3) crate
4) doggie psychologist

The most palatable and easiest option seemed to be a doggie run alongside the house. One gate already existed and I would hire my assistant's brother, Mark, to build another. In the interim (when Barry was speaking to me again), we barricaded the back patio French doors and decided we would leave the side garage door opened so Sparky could have shade and food indoors and be free to go in the backyard as well, when we weren't home.

This scheme worked for two days. Making my routine call home, I was told that Sparky was "at it" again. This time, the molding around the door from the garage to the house interior was ripped asunder. In addition, the mat in front of the door was in shreds and the bottom of the door evidenced a great deal of nail activity.

Without hesitation, I announced my intent to go to Petco for a crate. I was incredulous when Barry just agreed rather than suggest that Sparky might not be in the right place. A bullet dodged!

I purchased a large metal crate so that Sparky could see his surroundings from all sides. We put the crate in the garage. I placed an old, unwashed sweatshirt

73

of mine inside the crate to entice him in there, as it was now clear he was hopelessly infatuated with the woman of the house. After the first several days, Sparky knew the routine far too well and when crate time arrived, he would lie down and have to be dragged into what I had hoped would be his secure, safe, comforting daytime habitat. The next attempt at providing our anxious dog with a comfortable environment while we were out, was to bring the large, ugly, metallic crate into the kitchen where Sparky could be surrounded by the sights and smells of the pack. (I was doing lots of separation anxiety reading). Within a few weeks, Sparky had shown HIS metal. He had sprung several wires free from their molded joints, cut his paws and teeth in the process, and worked himself up to countless frenzies in the cage interior before I even left the house. So…we were on to a new, stronger cage and the doggie tranquilizer, Clomicalm. Now I HAD to make him love his daytime home, or else.

One evening after the boys went to bed, I set out to prove to Sparky that the crate was a good place to be. I crawled inside and lay with my head at the far end of the crate. I cooed, I said how wonderful it was—what a beautiful home—anything to convince Sparky he should LOVE it there. I lay there quietly looking through the crate at the ceiling thinking I must have totally, once and for all, lost my faculties. Soon thereafter, Sparky came in the cage. Of course, there wasn't room for the two of us and as I attempted to extricate myself, I prayed fervently Barry wouldn't come downstairs to investigate the commotion.

Well…another cage simply meant there was more steel to bend. We gave up on this one within a few weeks and just before his first anniversary with us, Sparky was left to his own devices—free inside the house—whenever we weren't home. Thankfully, that suited him just fine. There was daily evidence he tried every couch, chair, bed, and pillow just like Goldilocks, but apparently, he enjoyed the freedom, since he was not destructive. Drugged… but not destructive. By that time, Barry was Sparky's favorite back scratcher and often took him on evening walks. He'd never admit it, but Sparky won over Barry's heart as well (sort of).

Meaghan's only disappointment regarding Sparky was that the family didn't get a dog until she was away at college. Nevertheless, her breaks and summer vacations were a bonus for Sparky since he managed to attach himself to her whenever she was around. Michael often jokes that Sparky sought out his room only in desperation. It's true…he definitely favored the females. Nevertheless, the prettiest yellow lab ever, was part of the fabric of the household. And, as Michael's seizures worsened, Sparky's attentiveness to him increased.

For me, in addition to being the object of his unconditional love and devotion, Sparky provided essential distraction. Worries about Sparky's separation anxiety, thyroid dysfunction, arthritis, and cataracts occupied a part of my psyche that, at least temporarily, couldn't be utilized to invent worrisome scenarios involving Michael. Sparky provided not only welcome, but necessary, diversion. He loved and was loved in return. He came to the right place at the right time and lived out his cloudy-eyed days with his ill-suited name and his not very canine savvy family.

Sparky clearly was not seven at the time we adopted him. We guess now he must have been about nine. After he'd been with us just about four years, his hindquarters would collapse on our neighborhood walks about twice a week. Gradually, collapses became a daily occurrence, along with more frequent instances of incontinence and the occasional vomiting episode. None of our measures, including more frequent vet visits, seemed to improve Sparky's failing body systems. A dramatic fall downstairs early one December morning defined our next action. The kids said their final goodbyes at the house and Barry and I brought Sparky to the vet for the last time on December 4, 2004, the day before Michael's 20th birthday. Michael noted that it was okay to do so *then,* since his one wish for Sparky, to "make it through" Thanksgiving, had been realized.

Thanks, Sparky. RIP.

"You may have to fight a battle more than once to win it." —*Margaret Thatcher*

Keto Days

The final day of Michael's sophomore year was marked by a plane trip to San Jose, then onto Santa Cruz in a rental van, to begin our task of packing up Meaghan's belongings from her campus apartment and returning with her via a leisurely trip down the coast. The plane ride was uneventful if I don't account for the fact we three were the last on the plane and we ended up in the final two rows which face one another in this particular Southwest airplane. My flying nerves are generally in a pretty frayed state, and facing in the opposite direction in which the plane was traveling ranks among the most discomforting feelings I have had while aloft. Flight jitters aside, we arrived safely in San Jose, picked up our car, and got to the campus in time to treat Meaghan and her available roommates to dinner. It was a nice night...good food, wine, and company, and while Michael was not especially outgoing or talkative, that was easily chalked up to the strain of final exam week.

As we packed up Meaghan's belongings the following day, I thought to myself that Michael didn't seem quite "with it." Again, I attributed that to the stress of final exams and figured he would be more himself after a day or two. We left Santa Cruz mid-afternoon to begin what we thought of as a mini-vacation to celebrate the end of our sophomores' school years. Our first evening, we stopped at The Ragged Point Inn. We had a nice meal at the Big Sur lodging, (the wafting scent of Michael's chicken-rosemary pasta was headily apparent throughout the meal). Once, during dinner, he seemed to slam his water glass on the table. Since none of us actually saw a seizure motion, we couldn't be sure. But, the sinking feeling in my belly caused me to think that seizures might be on the increase again. After dinner, we wandered the grounds, taking in the spectacular coastline. We went to bed early so we'd beat the morning traffic on the treacherous two-lane coastal road. Michael had several brief tonic seizures during the night while asleep, but that was fairly typical of his seizure pattern then. We breakfasted at the lodge and then, as planned, got on the road early.

Michael and Meaghan were in the back seat; each frequently nodding off once we were beyond the scenic sights of Big Sur and the phenomenal spectacle of the elephant seals at San Simeone. We heard and observed Michael having a tonic seizure that lasted fifteen to twenty seconds, then...another...another... and another. He had about six to seven in a row before Barry was able to pull over to the side of the road. Michael was dazed, confused, belligerent, and pretty out of it. Once we thought the tonic activity had abated, we drove to a gas station and placed a call to Dr. Nespeca. He advised giving Michael an extra dose of one of his meds and to keep driving if we didn't feel it was yet an emergent experience. We cancelled our overnight Santa Monica plans and made the remaining five-hour trip in about four, without incident.

That evening, as I watched Michael swinging a baseball bat in the back yard, I discussed our options with Dr. Nespeca on the phone. He mentioned we might want to try a new drug called Keppra. It had been shown to be highly effective in people with Michael's seizure types. It would mean that, for a while, Michael would be on four anti-seizure meds as we increased the Keppra and tapered another down. I looked with marvel at our son who was out of it only hours before. Now, he was calling balls and strikes, imagining base hits and catches...providing quite an interesting play-by-play description. I marveled, too, that he seemed so limber and agile after so many muscle-tensing tonic seizure episodes. What should we do? Were things worsening enough to indicate a new drug should be tried? If we held off beginning the new drug until things got worse, we'd still be adjusting meds as Michael started the school year. THAT seemed to be a pattern. So...in spite of our resistance to ratcheting up medications or adding yet another, we decided to give this new, possible wonder drug, a try.

A few days after our return, my friend Anna gave me some information about herbs. In particular, she told me that rosemary might have some relation to seizures or the worsening of seizures. I did not do extensive research regarding whether this was indeed factual. I remembered only the strong rosemary-scented pasta at Ragged Point and I immediately pulled up our shrub in the backyard and banned Michael from eating the fabulous rosemary rolls at Pizza Nova. Small sacrifice, I thought, in view of the potential damage.

By Michael's first day of school, the Keppra dose was at the maximum he could have and we were slowly decreasing another med. He was, in a word, drugged. He attended classes, did assignments, and went to the special learning center on campus for tutorial help and to complete tests with extra time. Thankfully, THIS school really did try to honor student's individualized education plans.

The second week of school, Barry attended Parent's Night and had an opportunity to meet all of Michael's teachers. Afterward, Michael was upstairs doing homework while Barry and I had a late dinner. Upon my relentless querying, Barry uncharacteristically remarked that Michael had two female teachers he could only describe as "hardass."

During our first parent-teacher conference with Madeline in attendance several weeks later, we would learn just how hardass these ladies could be. The English teacher who I will refer to simply as Ms. B. (for b----) gave Michael a zero for the paper he turned in about his summer reading book because he hadn't made corrections to his first draft. He received no credit for reading the book (we had been thrilled with that accomplishment) and zero credit for the first draft, which was typed and, in our opinion, was a really good piece of work. I felt pretty justified in arguing (trying, trying, trying so hard to be cool and calm) for partial credit. I lost. Michael's grade at this point in time was a whopping fourteen percent.

Ms. B. couldn't let it go at that. Instead, she continued speaking and told us that she and Ms. W., (Barry's other "hardass") who was not present, determined based upon their review of Michael's admission data, that he should not be at the school. Oh dear...at that point, I thought Madeline was going to crawl across the broad conference table and wring Ms. B's neck. I was ALMOST amused by the image. In the meantime, though, Ms. B. managed to grab my attention as she related to other teachers that Michael would be on one page when the class was turning to another and though he followed directions, he did it "soooooooooo slowly."

I took that opportunity to inform the group that they were indeed seeing a dulled, slower, version of our son and that an EEG was being conducted that week to determine if the new drug regimen or additional seizures were the culprit. Could they please work with him till we get over this hurdle, I asked. Everyone, including Michael's assigned guidance counselor, and of course, except Ms. B. and undoubtedly, Ms. W., agreed. There was also agreement that any seizure activity that was observed would be reported either to the school nurse or to me via e-mail. At the time, tonic seizures were occurring in the daytime several times a week often with such force they could cause a fall or would cause objects held in Michael's hands to fall. The seizures generally lasted five seconds or less and Michael was clear (relatively) afterwards. I demonstrated the motions and the sounds and gave the usual "in the event of a seizure" speech. There were a few questions but everyone seemed comfortable with that aspect. I told them we would inform them of the EEG results and that we'd let them know of any changes to Michael's medications or seizure pattern. I asked again that they please do the same, noting that we could only act to change meds or actions if we were aware of seizures when they occured.

I felt pretty lousy after that meeting. It was a tough start to the year, which Michael could hardly afford. On the other hand, I felt his counselor, learning center teacher, and a couple of his teachers were very supportive and caring. I was afraid of the Misses B. and W. Madeline wasn't very happy after the meeting and passed some comments along to the principal regarding Ms. B.'s reporting of admission office information. When Madeline sought to get Michael transferred to another English class, she met no resistance at all.

The EEG revealed that the drug rather than absence seizures was the culprit. So...with another miracle drug deemed useless in our son's case, we were at yet another crossroad. What could we do? Dr. Nespeca reasoned that at age sixteen, with the desire to remain at his current school, Michael might be sufficiently motivated to try the highly restrictive ketogenic diet (think more restrictive than the strictest Atkins, all day, every day). We discussed it with Michael and he was all for trying "whatever" might help reduce his seizures and his medications. Michael and I met with the hospital dietician. Michael was the first Children's Hospital patient to be placed on the diet outside the inpatient setting. I was pleased that they had enough confidence in Michael to deal with the initial side effects and stick to it, and with me to put the right meal plan together to achieve a ketotic state which hopefully would reduce Michael's seizures and the need for some of his medications.

Barry and I read as much as we could about the diet. It has been used as a seizure treatment for many years. Meryl Streep even made a TV movie featuring the diet called *First Do No Harm*. The exact reason the diet is effective in reducing seizures in around thirty percent of the individuals on it, is not known. I had hoped to see a higher success rate but we were already pretty used to the law of thirds as it applied to most treatments: a third of the individuals get better, a third get worse, a third stay the same. Damn. Oh well...ANYTHING with any possibility to improve Michael's quality of life was always a go for us.

The dietician gave us a meal plan system, outlining by grams the amount of fat, protein, and carbohydrates Michael could have throughout the day. There were very few carbohydrate grams allowed. An incredibly high amount of fat grams were required including those obtained through an oil known as MCT oil, and small though fairly reasonable portions of protein could be consumed. We were informed Michael probably wouldn't gain weight. Most likely, his already skeletal frame would feature even more boney prominences. We also were aware that when his system was becoming ketotic he could experience nausea, vomiting, diarrhea, and cramping. He was game, so we moved on.

Barry and I began the Atkins diet so that our evening meals were quite close to what Michael was eating. We ordered an Atkins bread mix on the Internet. Barry made it weekly in our bread machine and we learned to slice it thinly enough to amount to six grams worth of bread for Michael's packed lunch each day. His carb allowance was generally between twenty to twenty-five grams per day. It is absolutely AMAZING how many foods contain carbs. I became a vigilant label reader and made a pretty good tomato sauce with very little tomato.

With the exception of viewing Michael retching and vomiting about two nights a week, the diet days were pretty positive for an extended period of time. Michael grew more alert, and by the spring of his junior year, we were able to start decreasing his Topamax. What a difference! There he was again... more alert, humorous, social, and happier. Michael has a terrific smile. It takes over his face and exudes a confidence that is often absent from his life. We were seeing it more and more and enjoying every moment. It was obvious, too, that he was developing friendships. He had an occasional movie outing and on days we picked him up at school, he would often be talking with girls who became if not friends, at least caring classmates. The seeming success of the diet made the non-reporting of daytime classroom seizures by the teachers a little easier to handle. I still steam though, about the time Ms. W. said, "God bless you" when during a brief tonic seizure, Michael fell on his backpack in a classroom aisle. When I asked why she did this, her response was, "So he wouldn't be embarrassed." She rendered me speechless.

Michael didn't complain too much while he was on the diet. He grew to accept that it could be the ticket to fewer seizures and less medication and he was faithful to following through with the requirements every day. We really admired his determination and dedication.

Schoolwork was, as always, a struggle. But at least Michael was getting by. Our goal was crystal clear. graduation. Junior year was almost a wrap and it seemed like it was the best year of the last few. As summer neared, the Connolly household dared to be optimistic.

"Be courageous. It's one of the only places left uncrowded." —*Anita Roddick*

Hanging by a Thread

My late father's words sit in the forefront of my sleepless night's thoughts, "Hang tough, Mary Lou."

"Sure Dad," I think, "but it was a lot easier to do that when you were here reminding me." I'm TRYING to hang tough, but the harder I try, it seems even worse things happen. Once we think we've experienced the worst yet, it gets worse still. I lay in bed talking to my father and in a rare commune with God, cursing the fate that has befallen us. I am not in a good place. When people ask me how I am, I'm actually telling them I'm "hanging by a thread." Some hanging tough, huh, Daddy!

It's May 28, 2002 and my cell phone rings. "Mrs. Connolly, it's Deb, the nurse at school. Michael's had a seizure."

"A grand mal?" I ask incredulously. (This hasn't ever occurred in school.)

"Yes, we called the paramedics and they're now here."

"He's responding now, what do you want us to do?"

"I'll come for him," I say, knowing that a trip to the emergency room is simply going to be a waste of time and money.

"No," Deb replies after checking with the paramedics, "since he's not eighteen, they'll need to take him to the hospital."

I replied quickly, "Okay, I'll meet them at Children's."

"Children's?" she asked.

My firm and insistent response, "Yes, Children's is where his neurologist practices." Then, I had one more question now that I knew Michael was waking up. "Was he incontinent?"

Deb responded with a simple, "No."

I breathed a sigh of relief. At least he wouldn't have to deal with that.

I arrived at the emergency room and was directed to a three-bed room off the nurses' station. Poking out the end of the third curtain was a familiar pair of hairy legs and sneakers. Michael was sitting on the stretcher laughing and chatting it up with the nurse. The nurse, Carol, much to my relief and comfort, had been a colleague of mine at the academic teaching hospital that had closed both our departments in the prior year. First, hugs and kisses to Michael, then, to Carol, who pretty much reiterated what I was thinking, "WHY is he HERE?" This visit would be our briefest of the following six months. Oh, if we only knew what was ahead, what then?

Meaghan returned from college to spend the summer in San Diego during the second week of June. Michael was in the middle of finals week and I was concerned about how stressed out he seemed. Barry and I comforted ourselves with the explanation that to be stressed he must be more "with it" in terms of the importance of exam grades. Michael took an early morning shower on the day of his math exam. Per the usual routine, Barry was in the kitchen preparing Michael's lunch and I was getting dressed to go to work (closing my department) before I came downstairs to make Michael's breakfast.

Suddenly, there was a thud in the bathroom. I raced in and found Michael in the throes of a seizure, his head wedged between the hard marble shower stall and the side of the toilet. His gangly, naked body lay half on the bathmat stretched across the stone floor, stiffening and jerking. I screamed Barry's name but he was already upstairs in response to the crash of body against floor. Meaghan had made it to the bathroom at the same time I did and she was pretty much freaking out as well. Our highly controlled responses to Michael's seizures were a thing of the past. I, no better than she, sat perched on the toilet seat desperately trying to protect Michael's head from incurring any more injury that it may have received from the fall. My fear was that if he stopped breathing, he would do so out of reach of his mother's arms on the cold, hard surface we had just installed and I now hated! Barry brought some level of calm to the scene. He took my place on the seat and when Michael's body began to relax he eased his torso up out of the cramped space.

I cradled his head in my lap, "It's okay, Mike; it'll be okay. Can you hear me, Michael?"

In the meantime, Meaghan reached the neurologist on-call who instructed us to call 9-1-1 because of the potential head injury. We lifted Michael to his bed, and he helped us help him into a pair of flannel PJ bottoms and we awaited the arrival of the San Diego Fire Department paramedics. The paramedics were preceded by a fire truck, so even at the early hour, the commotion at the Connolly household was witnessed by a few neighbors. Six men and women filed up the stairs, kindly did not chastise the nurse-mother for moving Michael, examined him in his bed, then placed him in a special carrier to get him downstairs. Then, they transferred him to the more familiar stretcher, and placed him in the back of the ambulance. The firemen and paramedics during this and all subsequent encounters were competent, considerate, and in many instances, highly compassionate. I thought them all worthy of being in my father's esteemed profession.

I rode in the front of the ambulance to Children's where I entered more somberly than at the prior visit since THIS time I felt we needed to be there. Meaghan and Barry drove to the hospital in Barry's car. I looked for and found Carol's friendly face upon our arrival and she promptly ministered to Michael (AND Mom). Meaghan and Barry arrived and we sat like three sad lumps awaiting the visit of the on-call neurologist. I think we were all shocked by the incident. We recognized now that a fall could happen anyplace, anytime. Of course, we really knew this all along, but denial, it turns out, is quite a useful coping mechanism. We knew we might not be there the next time to cushion and to comfort. A bleak reality was setting in. Dr. Schultz recommended we increase the Topamax dose slightly. We had been highly resistant to this suggestion after the first seizure, since we had almost totally weaned Michael OFF Topamax during the seeming success of the ketogenic diet. Now, of course, it was a different story. We simply couldn't have Michael seizing and falling every two weeks.

We went home scarred and scared. Meaghan still cannot sleep whenever Michael showers. She leaves her room that is adjacent to the bathroom and lies in wait in another room until he opens the bathroom door towel-clad and safely out. For months, I couldn't be further than ten feet from the bathroom when he was in it. In the six months after the bathroom incident, I must have knocked and asked, "Are you okay?" hundreds of times. It is still positively, absolutely the worst part of the day. This routine activity, this daily occurrence, has caused a disproportionate amount of angst—not to mention the annoyance it causes Michael! How tolerant he has been of our overbearing zeal to keep him from harm. How dare I become annoyed at my mother during a visit when she points out how long he's been in the bathroom! Yes, here we all are—hanging by a thread!

Fast forward to December. By my calculation, every eight to fourteen days, Michael has had a major seizure event since the end of May. Several occurred at home and though frightening, we managed to control them afterwards with Valium. If the incidents occurred at school, we met the paramedics at the emergency room. All told, there were five more ambulance trips from the high school campus to Children's Hospital from May to December. Michael was very, very busy just trying to stay upright and thanks to increasing doses of seizure meds, also trying to maintain some semblance of alertness. Progress was occurring, but definitely not in the direction we wanted.

On December 3rd, I answered my cell phone. A frantic voice identifying itself as a secretary at the high school told me she was asked to call and tell me Michael had a seizure and he was at the "bottom of the senior stairs." She could not answer if he fell down the stairs but volunteered there was "lots of blood" and the paramedics were on the way. I told her I'd meet the ambulance at the emergency room and I would contact Barry to do the same. I called the school on the way to the hospital. This time, the voice on the other end could tell me Michael was conscious. When I was then connected to the nurse, Deb used words that indicated Michael was in an agitated state. She reported he did have some facial and head wounds which "looked like a lot of blood to a lay person" and that he was in the hands of the paramedics. Later, as Barry and I waited in the ambulance bay at the hospital, Deb called us to report Michael had "calmed down a lot" but we should be aware he'd look "pretty restrained" when we saw him.

Since Barry and I made it to the emergency room long before the ambulance arrived, I entered the waiting area and caught the eye of a nurse who was on duty during a prior ER visit. The nurse gave me the initial paperwork to complete, directed us to the area where the ambulance would arrive (we knew of course, since this was now somewhat of a routine), and checked on us periodically as we must have LOOKED like we felt—defeated, worn, frazzled, terrified. Things simply could not continue this way.

Though the school nurse had tried to prepare us, we still weren't ready for the sight of our son. The paramedics assured us he was "recovering" as they prepared to move him into the emergency room. Michael was taped to the stretcher from the tip of his head to his toes. The tape across his forehead wasn't quite covering an egg-sized purple/pink mass of skin that was lacerated the length of it and bleeding slightly. His nose oozed blood and beneath it on the right side a gash was somewhat visible underneath congealed blood and above a lip now swollen to three times normal size. A smaller gash on the bridge of his nose had clotted nicely and the tip of his nose was sporting an abrasion that must have occurred prior to the act of the kindly teacher who placed his own shirt under Michael's face to minimize the trauma of the seizure. He was a mess. He was also still somewhat agitated I noted, as he nearly broke my fingers when I tried to hold his hand. I thought to myself at that point that it would not be easy for the school to have him back. There would be worry that in the post-seizure state such as he was in today, he could harm himself or others. I dismissed the thought to deal with it later and focused on the present: banged up kid with obvious trauma to the head. I would press for an X-ray. No need. The sweet attending physician, whose looks and actions reminded us of Meaghan, ordered a neck X-ray and a CT scan.

After the neck X-ray was read as negative, the neck brace was removed. Michael appeared more comfortable then and far less agitated. After several hours, Barry asked if someone could clean Michael's wounds. Another doctor told him that the cuts and abrasions were not their primary concern but nonetheless he sent in an aide who proceeded to wipe Michael's wounds with a facecloth she dipped in the top of a hydrogen peroxide bottle. My thoughts as she wiped, dipped, wiped, dipped, and wiped again were that I just didn't feel this was the most sanitary and effective way to cleanse his wounds. But, in my altered state, I chose not to voice my concerns. Following the "cleansing," a CT scan was performed. The results would be read within a half-hour we were told, and then, the attending physician who took over from Meaghan's look-a-like at change of shift, would contact Dr. Nespeca regarding Michael's meds. By then, it was dark outside and still no medication had been administered for seizures. (Michael had been having very slight twitching, jerking ones ever since his arrival.) The CT scan result was negative and I watched and listened as the emergency attending MD relayed information to Dr. Nespeca fully knowing that the phone would eventually be in my hands. At one point, I overheard him say, "No, he hasn't had any seizures since being here."

To which I said, "Yes, he has had many small ones and just minutes ago had a tonic which lasted about ten seconds."

The ER doctor then said, "Well, Mom says he's had some but since I did not witness them, I can only report what she's telling me."

Then, the phone was handed to me per Dr. Nespeca's request and he I discussed medication options. The plan was made and revised several times during our conversation. In the end, the agreement was to increase the Topamax dosage rapidly—every two days we would increase the dose by 50 milligrams until we reached 500 milligrams per day. In the past, we had increased Topamax by 25 milligrams per week! We knew we could expect to see more significant side effects including drowsiness, speech-finding difficulties, and certainly heightened irritability, but we hoped most would be transient.

Now, all that needed to be done was to suture Michael's gashes. It was already after six so I requested that Michael's evening meds be ordered from the pharmacy and given. That accomplished, I left the hospital to check on Sparky and order some food for when the guys arrived home. I was happy to leave Barry to watch the suturing. I can't explain why I couldn't bear to watch. I just knew it might send me over the edge and I wasn't ready to go there.

On the way home, I reflected on the day's events, trying to spin a positive out of it. Well...he didn't get seriously injured. AND his friends from school came to see him in the ER. Though she informed us it was normally not "policy" to let teen friends in, the receptionist was so impressed with "nice boys" like Evan and Will, that she allowed them entrance. THAT was really heartwarming. What else? It appeared that with a day of rest or two Michael would be back in the thick of things on campus.

Sparky met me in the pitch-black house and nudged my legs until he felt he hadn't REALLY been deserted. I then ordered far too much food from a local restaurant that delivered and settled back to await Barry's and Michael's arrival home.

The food was delivered and the boys showed up within moments after. We were eating quietly when the phone rang. Barry answered. It was Meaghan. On our end, I heard questions and commands.

"Where will you stay? Call when you get there."

Barry handed me the phone. Meaghan was laughing as she said, "Dad's being weird."

"Why do you say that?" I asked.

She told me that instead of driving directly from Santa Cruz to Del Mar the next day as planned, she and her friends were going to go as far as Santa Barbara and stay with friends. "Oh, that's why Dad was giving you the business." Continuing the charade, I asked a few questions about the "boys" these twenty-one year old young women were going to see. She hung up happy and blissfully ignorant of the chaos on the home front. I was relieved. Michael's face would have another day to heal before his sister laid her eyes on it.

I slept in the trundle in Michael's room that night. I was less concerned about seizures than I was the fact he'd incurred a head injury and I wanted to be sure there were no symptoms of trouble gone unnoticed. The night was uneventful; that being, Michael slept peacefully; I awoke at every snore, toss, and turn.

I didn't think it possible, but Michael's face looked even worse the following morning. It was hurtful to behold. Other than grogginess and slowness to respond that could be attributed to the seizures, head trauma, and increase in medication, Michael seemed to be in reasonable shape.

I, on the other hand, was in the most fragile of states. I spoke early in the morning with my friend Anna who called to check in on us. I assured her we were OK, sincerely meaning it at that moment. Soon thereafter, my next caller was Michael's guidance counselor from high school. I was rattling on about when Michael could probably return, homework assignments Barry could pick-up, and so on, when he ever so gently suggested we think about an alternative schooling arrangement until Michael's condition was "stabilized." I can't account for WHY the conversation so totally unraveled me. It isn't as if I hadn't had the thought the high school would be hesitant about having him back, or that we hadn't recognized he was falling further and further behind in his classroom work. All I know is that I told the counselor to look into the alternative he suggested and get back to me. I hung up. I fell to pieces. From then on, with the exception of the return call from Michael's counselor, I could not make it through any conversation that day with anyone (aunt, president of investment club, former secretary, business partner and friend) without weeping disconsolately. I was at the lowest point ever and didn't care who knew it. A turning point of sorts, I guess.

I called Barry at work, again unable to put two sentences together without quietly wailing, and told him he HAD to tie up the loose ends at the high school since I (obviously) was unable to conduct an appropriate conversation. I know I worried him, but again, I couldn't will myself to "be strong" or "hang tough" at that particular point.

By mid-afternoon, I had recovered most of my composure and felt better because we now had a plan for Michael's schooling as well as his future treatment. I resolved to go forward with my plan to attend the epilepsy fundraising event, Gingerbread City, with my friends Suzanne and Anna. I felt infinitely better once I showered and primped myself up to an acceptable cocktail party look. Barry arrived home to spend the evening with a mellow but more alert Michael. After Suzanne inspected Michael's wounds and suggested a three-time-a-day swabbing with peroxide and application of an antibacterial ointment, we were off to the event.

I heard from a number of people that it looked like I was "having a ball" that night. I was. I wasn't. While true that red wine dulled my immediate concerns, Michael was "there" in every way. Early in the evening, I locked eyes with another member of the Epilepsy Foundation Board. She had lost a son to epilepsy complications eighteen months earlier. Call it woman's intuition or even more particularly, the intuition of a mother of a child with seizures, Sue read in that one glance the pain I could not cover up with my sparkling emerald earrings, lacy black blouse, or Christmas-red lips. She saw, I knew…and I couldn't speak to her. To do so, I would have broken the make-believe aura I had wrapped myself in to keep the seizure demons away for a few fleeting hours. How could I fa-la-la and schmooze for the Epilepsy Foundation if I was pouring my heart out to a mom who was trying to get through another holiday season without her beloved son? Later that week, I received a note from Sue telling me I'd been on her mind since that evening. I marveled at her ability to reach out to me in the midst of her own anguish. I even felt a bit guilty… "At least I still have MY Michael," I thought.

Meaghan arrived home for Christmas break the following day. Michael and I greeted her at the door. She stared at her brother's battered face. The egg on his forehead was yellowing and his lip was swollen to twice its normal size—he looked a LOT better to me, but to her, he looked simply dreadful. After she took the scene in, we told her when the incident occurred and how we decided not to tell her so she'd enjoy her Santa Barbara detour. She was grateful we had kept that little secret from her and worried that the battle to achieve seizure control was, at this point, being won by the seizure side. I was grateful she hadn't been around the previous day since it allowed me the time to emote unfettered by concern regarding the effect my behavior might have on her.

The additional recovery day also brought new energy and determination to my desire to arrange the Vagus Nerve Stimulator implant for Michael post haste. Meaghan, on the other hand, needed some adjustment time of her own. For the next few days, she would isolate herself from her friends and wrap herself in the cocoon of family; however fractured and fragile that family was at the moment.

"Be patient. Our prayers are always answered, but not always on the exact date we want them to be." —*Marjorie Turner*

The Last Semester

I was, quite honestly, a woman possessed. I was adamantly opposed to Dr. Nespeca's suggestion to place Michael on a drug called Felbatol that previously had failed to control his seizures. Since his seizures began, Michael had been on about a dozen drugs. Enough!

For years, I had erroneously believed Michael was not a candidate for the Vagus Nerve Stimulator (VNS). The VNS is a device that transmits electrical impulses to the brain from a pacemaker implanted in the chest by way of the left vagus nerve. It reduces seizure frequency, intensity and duration.

During the days immediately following Michael's most catastrophic seizure on school grounds, I read everything I could get my hands on about the VNS device. I called the local representative of the company which made the VNS, to obtain a video and the company-produced literature. We all watched the video and read the pamphlets and other materials which explained how this pacemaker implant worked and how its use had changed numerous patients' lives because it helped control their seizures and enabled many of them to reduce their medications. The video was slick, and the literature obviously touted the patient successes while in finer print the old rule of thirds was mentioned; a third of the patients obtain "dramatic improvement" in seizure control, a third experience "good improvement", another third experience "little or no improvement." Out of options because a new miracle medication did not exist, and increasing the meds Michael was on would only send him into a deeper haze-like state, we made a decision in concert with Dr. Nespeca to try something new.

Michael was fully on board with the decision to insert the VNS, and I quickly navigated through the insurance and scheduling maze with the assistance of Lisa, the upbeat and energetic Cyberonics sales rep who also happened to be a nurse. Michael was scheduled for the outpatient procedure on December 18, during school's Christmas break. He was finishing up his first semester work at a private, independent high school which he attended once weekly for meetings with his teachers to review the five to six hours of home study he did for each of the courses. This system worked well with one glaring exception: he had little or no peer interaction and felt isolated. He was anxious to get back to his campus school site and that was a motivator to perform to the best of his ability and to get on with the process of VNS insertion.

My mom arrived for her winter stay in mid-December. Normally, I would spare her the details of the surgical procedure until it was safely accomplished, but her travel plans had been made long before Michael's most traumatic fall and injuries earlier in the month. His face had a couple of weeks to heal before her arrival, but the scars and redness that remained, were enough to convince her we needed to take the slight risks involved in VNS implantation in order to achieve the potential positive outcome. So it was that we were celebrating her birthday at Jake's on the evening before Michael's surgery, and he chowed down in anticipation of the fast he would have to keep after midnight. It was a fun evening. We all knew Grammie's wish as she blew out the candle on her Mud Pie.

Michael was an "add-on" surgical case, meaning his case would start after the neurosurgeon's final case of the day was completed. We left the house mid-afternoon to begin the pre-operative procedures at Children's Day Surgery Center. It was a long wait and I worried more about Meaghan and my mother worrying at home, than I did about the procedure itself. (We are genetically linked and challenged by our capacity to worry). I had every confidence in Dr. Levy since he taught other surgeons how to do the procedure, and he had inserted a sufficient number of devices. In addition, I was able to secure the same anesthesiologist whom we entrusted Michael to on at least two prior occasions.

Michael's primary focus during the wait was his growling stomach. He'd only gone off the ketogenic diet a month earlier and he was in the midst of making up for lost carbs with a vengeance. His 5'7" frame at 116 pounds was quite thin. The surgery took less than an hour, and the half-inch disk placed in the left side was quite prominent in Michael's skeletal chest. I marveled at Dr. Levy's ability to sew the sparse patch of skin back together. We could view the suture line because an invisible glue-like "bandage" was all that covered it. The neck wound where the wires were manipulated around the left vagus nerve was covered with a dressing that I could change daily until we saw the surgeon the following week. Michael recovered well from the anesthesia, and a call home assured Meaghan and my Mom all was well and we'd join them shortly.

Michael's wounds healed without any complications. Dr. Levy sent us from our post-op visit with words to the effect he'd see Michael in about ten years (the average time to replace the pacemaker). Activating and programming the VNS was to occur in Dr. Nespeca's office in January. In the interim, Michael's seizures were non-existent; the same effect we'd noticed for a few weeks after he'd had any general anesthesia.

We truly enjoyed the holiday season. We had my mother and Meaghan with us for several weeks, Michael was on the mend surgically, and he had successfully not only completed the semester, but also achieved great grades at the alternative school. While proud of his ability to do that, he was most excited about the prospect of returning to his "real school" following the winter break. Barry and I were excited about the prospect that the VNS would help to improve the quality of Michael's life.

Michael returned to school in January and from all teachers' reports had a great first week back: "alert, attentive, personable, able to follow directions," were just a few of the descriptors we heard. We started to be cautiously optimistic. We certainly had experienced a good week or two *before*, that was forgotten in the chaos of a new crisis. But this time...maybe things would be different.

Things were different—but not in the way we'd hoped. During Michael's second week back at school, we received an e-mail from his anatomy and physiology teacher relating how he seemed "easily confused" and when she worked with him on an explanation, moments later it appeared he'd "totally forgotten" whatever was said. I trusted her judgment. She had been the one teacher who always kept us informed. She was great at assessing Michael's strengths and weaknesses and she had made learning more interesting for him. Armed with her comments and our own observations, I asked Dr. Nespeca to order an EEG. I was suspicious that Michael was experiencing another type of seizure: absence. I was familiar with them since he did have them years earlier but hadn't experienced this seizure type or been treated for them for several years. The EEG was performed while Michael was doing homework. It confirmed that indeed, he was having absence (formerly called petit mal) seizures for significant periods of time. Since the VNS was in the earliest stages of adjustment, Michael was placed on another med to control these seizures.

I called the school nurse the following day to inform her of the "new" seizure type, give information about how the seizures manifested and asked that teachers let her or Barry and I know if they suspected any activity. I was taken aback when she sighed and said she didn't think the teachers could handle any more activity to observe, and then she went on to say Michael should probably "have a full-time aide in the classroom in a public school," and that I should consider looking into that. I got the impression during our conversation that she was probably advising school management regarding the risks of keeping Michael on campus. Her mind was made up...it was simply too risky. Later that day, I talked with the school counselor and we discussed the possibility of Michael returning to the independent high school. He too, carefully chose words, but it was transparently clear that school administration was worried about liability. I simply didn't have the energy to fight them. The principal remained a strong advocate for Michael. He was a kind and caring man who assured us Michael would graduate with his class. I didn't want to make his life any more difficult. So...the life that would be made more difficult in this instance was my son's. Life sometimes sucks big time, I thought.

Michael was not a happy camper, but gamely attended his weekly teacher sessions and worked at least six hours every day on his subjects. For the first time in years, he had time to enjoy the evenings. It appeared to us that coursework actually could be accomplished during the course of a day. Hmmmm. Why is this not so in our public and private schools? Something's wrong with this picture, I noted. But I would not tackle this issue. We only had a few months till the ultimate goal, graduation, was reached. I was not about to rock any boats or rattle any education cages.

I was still consulting in the home health business and during the times I traveled, I made arrangements for Michael to spend his days at Suzanne's home with Mike, her husband, who is a stay-at-home Dad. It was good for my Michael to be out of his own house and Mike enjoyed the forays into anatomy and physiology because of his nurse anesthetist background. Getting Michael to focus was a challenge. He was now on high doses of three anti-seizure drugs. Mike was great about giving Michael breaks and doing a variety of activities to "perk him up." Educating Michael in the drugged state he was in, was definitely a group process.

The first week of February, I was booked for a job in Sacramento. The day before I was to leave, Michael called me into his bathroom while he showered. "Mom, come get all these ants on the wall." I climbed atop the toilet seat and was busy swiping a small army of ants when I heard the vocalization that often signaled the beginning of a tonic seizure.

"Oh, God, BAAAAARRY," I shrieked, as I opened the shower door determined to break Michael's fall. And, I did. I positioned myself behind him and in front of the marble bench seat, and we slid together as the shower pelted us both. Barry arrived in seconds, turned off the water, and watched helplessly as Michael seized in my arms. We waited a minute, maybe two, until the stiffening jerks subsided. Then, another few moments until he could be roused enough to be walked to his room and his bed where he would sleep soundly for several hours. I got out of my sopping PJs, sobbed a bit, checked on my peaceful son, said bye to Barry, and used the rest of the day to talk myself into continuing on with the week as planned. Poor Barry. What a sight we must have been. It was like slapstick comedy without the laugh track.

The next day, I was sporting huge bruises on both arms and one of my hind cheeks was covered in the most ghastly purple. That one hurt but not nearly as much as the unspoken thought, "What if the VNS doesn't work?"

I went to Sacramento as planned and was assured each evening that all was well at home. Michael seemed back to baseline when we spoke. It was good to have a job to focus on. Good for all of us!

Sometime in April, we received something in the mail from the high school. It stated we should plan on attending an award ceremony in May because our child was receiving one. It was a generic note and I didn't pay too much attention but thought I should call to see if I really needed to change plans for a work-related trip. I couldn't fathom what the campus-absent senior would be awarded.

When I spoke to the administrative secretary she was very clear, "Yes, change your plans, Mrs. Connolly. There are only two people in the entire school receiving this award."

So, I re-scheduled.

On a beautiful, sunny, Sunday in May the high school gym was crammed for the ceremony. Michael seemed happy to be among his old classmates. We sat through what seemed several hours of scholarship awards. Later, much later, in the ceremony, they announced Michael's name as recipient of an award named after a faculty member. Michael slowly walked toward the stage to warm applause and a few scattered "go Mike" cheers. The award was to acknowledge great courage and perseverance in overcoming a significant obstacle. Were we proud? Of course. We knew all Michael had endured over the years. In addition to seizures, the snickers of classmates, the isolation, not being part of the "in" crowd, the lack of socialization, the constant, never-ending schooling, the hospital stays, the emergency transports from the high school campus, blood tests, IVs, the fog of medications, and the nausea and vomiting and cramping of ketosis to name a few. Yes, we knew and truly did appreciate the acknowledgement. Yet, it was a bittersweet moment. Michael would NOT return to this school the following day. Though commending his bravery, they were afraid to take him back on campus. So be it…award in hand, following the ceremony, we visited one of La Jolla's best restaurants, Roy's, for a Hawaii-inspired feast. Michael finished off his meal with a serving of dark, rich, chocolate fudge lava cake. Lots of carbs! All in all, a good day.

Michael was progressing well with the new education routine. Graduation was within his grasp. Meaghan too, was completing HER last semester at Santa Cruz. Though she was scheduled to graduate on June 14th and Michael on the 7th, she insisted on flying home between finals to attend, in her words, "the most important graduation." My mom planned to fly out from Massachusetts with Michael's godfather, my brother, Gary. The game plan was that Gary would attend Michael's graduation then spend a few days visiting with us. After Gary's departure back to Massachusetts, Michael, Grammie, Barry, and I would drive up the coast in two cars to pack Meaghan's belongings and attend her graduation. Then…on to Oahu, Hawaii for some seriously splendid R&R. As June neared, the anticipation in the household was palpable. What a relief it would be not to deal with formal education for a while. What a joy to have two graduates. What a milestone not to have had a significant daytime seizure episode since mid-February. Life was settling down a bit though we were ever mindful that could change in an instant.

Michael completed his finals in fine fashion assuring that he would indeed be able to graduate with his class. Gary, my mother, and Meaghan arrived as scheduled. I was caught up in planning a graduation party for Michael. His sole request: a karaoke machine so he could carry out his self-promise to sing in front of people as a step toward diminishing his public-speaking fears. (It wasn't REALLY a self-promise. He had actually bet Madeline he would sing "You've Lost that Lovin' Feeling" and she was planning to attend to see if he'd follow through.) I wanted an atmosphere that was simultaneously low-key and celebratory. Michael never liked a lot of fuss made over him for any reason. Though I felt we had reason to be dancing in the streets and shouting from the rooftops, instead, we'd gather with the close network of family and friends who'd been there for us throughout this journey.

Michael attended a practice session and picked up his cap and gown for the graduation ceremony. Finally, with the fire-engine red garments in his possession, it all began to seem real.

Graduation day was a cool June-gloom day with a wet drizzle falling, but nothing could dampen the spirits of the Connolly clan. This was IT! As soon as the first note sounded and the four hundred plus graduates started walking into the college gymnasium, my heart was in my throat and my eyes misted over. I was physically choking on sobs. When we spotted Michael, I became momentarily worse but managed to pull together quickly to savor every moment. The pictures afterward captured a handsome young man with an enormous grin and hugs for anyone close by, including a couple of very pretty graduates who singled him out and told him "I'll miss you". The camera captured a mosaic of relief, accomplishment, finality, and pride in all our faces. We would party the next day with family and friends. Today was a day to experience the fabulous food of Chef Bernard at the Marine Room in La Jolla with our small group. Chef Bernard and our waiter were very attentive, giving the graduate some special delicacies including a second dessert. Michael really did feel special and we did too, to share in his accomplishment.

The following day, Michael mingled and chatted with the guests at his party. Some people commented that he seemed more alert and was in good humor. He sang his song and collected from Madeline. He seemed relaxed. We were thrilled. We ALL needed a break from the grind of teaching/learning that had inhabited so many of our waking hours for so many years.

Meaghan returned to school the following day to take the last of her finals and gear up for her own graduation. We were very proud. She was getting her degree in four years from a UC school, she was applying to law schools, and she had emerged from four years at Santa Cruz, a beautiful, sensible, accomplished young woman.

Our trip up the coast to Santa Cruz was uneventful. My mother and I followed Barry and Michael and managed not to get separated for the seven-hour drive. We arrived when the sun was shining on the Santa Cruz wharf, just below our motel suite that included a private patio and hot tub. The price per night of our motel accommodations was more than we'd be paying the following week at the high-end Pink Palace in Oahu. However, we were used to the price gouging which occurred in this small college town during every orientation, parent, or graduation weekend. Nothing, not even outrageous price gouging, would put a crimp in the second leg of Connolly graduations.

The following day was glorious. There was a blue, cloudless sky, and the sun was shining brilliantly on Monterey Bay as we all prepared to go to the Merrill College ceremony scheduled for ten a.m. We were pleased that Merrill's was the first ceremony of the day, and that we would not be sitting on the athletic field in midday sun. As anticipated, the ceremony had an air of informality. The graduates sauntered past us often yelling back at or hugging vocal family members and friends. As each graduate accepted their diploma and walked across the stage, the kneeling family photographers traded spaces as if in a weird rendition of musical chairs. After a Bush-bashing speech that did not seem wholly appropriate for the occasion though certainly was in the Santa Cruz tradition, we met our grad and cleared the campus to allow for the next graduating college. We used the afternoon to lounge around and catch some rays (Barry, Michael, and my Mom) and to help Meaghan pack (me). Later, we had a special meal at a restaurant overlooking the boardwalk and broad expanse of beach. Graduation number two: mission accomplished.

We left early the next day, two cars packed full. Since we were leaving for Hawaii in a few days, we wanted to drive straight through to Del Mar. I wanted my mom to see Big Sur so we decided to take the coastal route. The drive was gorgeous as usual, but I was keenly disappointed my mother refused to look, since the height and proximity to the edge of the seaside cliffs pretty much terrified her. I gave her a lot of good-natured grief, as did Meaghan, but she stubbornly faced east until we arrived at sea level.

"Earth is crammed with heaven." —*Elizabeth Barrett Browning*

The Pleasure of Pink

The household was excited. In just a few days, we'd board a Hawaiian Airlines flight out of San Diego and land in bustling Oahu. I was probably the one most eagerly anticipating the trip because I was the planner. Over the years, vacation planning became a way for me to escape the day-to-day events of life be they routine or catastrophic, and to imagine the sights, smells, and textures of unvisited places before we ever landed. Generally, I was pretty adept at this planning thing, utilizing a variety of guidebooks and Internet reviews. Because I am an unabashed foodie, restaurant choices are based on my knowledge of a chef's background and the contents of his/her cookbook(s). I did rely on a travel agent to guide me through my choice between The Royal Hawaiian Hotel (affectionately known as the Pink Palace) OR a five-star hotel along the same Waikiki beachfront. The agent said that the Royal Hawaiian had an old-time Hawaii feel, especially if we requested a stay in the historic wing. Since we'd already heard almost the exact words from our friend Don Tremblay and I am more inclined toward warm and cozy than austere, I opted for pink. My brother Gerry, still unattached at the time, was going to fly in from Chicago and meet us in Honolulu. In the early stages of the planning phase, I booked two rooms, figuring guys in one and girls in the other. Then, most importantly, I contacted the hotel's delightful concierge, Wendy, and told her my restaurant choices. She exclaimed she couldn't have done better and told me to leave the reservations in her hands. She promptly called me to confirm everything and I told her I'd be sure to see her at check-in.

The flight to the island was smooth and at five hours, seemed short, too. Gerry's flight arrived within moments of ours and we crammed everyone into a mini-van and drove through the busy city until we veered off just a few yards and pulled up to heaven on earth. As I entered the lobby, I was struck by the aqua color of the water that caught my eye to the right. I went to the desk to check in. The rest of my party was lured closer to the beckoning ocean. When I asked if there was an opportunity for an upgrade, I was told that had already been accomplished. Six of us entered the historic wing and our suite-like rooms. Barry and I took the king-size bedroom; Michael would occupy the pull-out couch just beyond a set of French doors. Meaghan and my mom took the double beds in the adjoining room with Gerry's sleeping quarters designated the pull-out sofa in their suite space. This was an unexpected beginning to a restful, re-invigorating, healing, hopeful week.

Ask me about any of our prior vacations and I'll speak mostly in generalities about what was nice, where we went, what we ate, etc. However, this vacation, Oahu, I can see, smell, touch, and taste. There was the warmth and beauty of the water with the large but gentle wave swells that both Michael and my mother could easily romp in with no worries of riptides or undertows. Then, there was the image of my mom's straw hat bobbing above the waves shielding her from the sun and distressingly, fading the Phil Mickelson autograph she obtained in Hartford one year. We looked forward to daily breakfasts in the bountiful buffet of the Surf restaurant...mmmm; made to order eggs, waffles, smoothies, and the freshest of fruit, the best Kona coffee, the most polite wait staff. Pink lounge chairs covered with pink towels awaited us each day in the pink roped-in area of the most beautiful stretch of Waikiki Beach. We took our lunch break at the beachside café and enjoyed the great local beer and sandwiches and goodies for sharing. We gathered for tropical cocktails in the same café post-shower and pre-dinner. We even got my mom to try the special Mai tai, supposedly invented in this very place. The restaurant choices were on the mark. Each dinner experience was better than the night before... though all were outstanding for different reasons. We simply couldn't go wrong anywhere. Michael's goal appeared to be to try a new fish entrée each night. My mother's eyes were wide with disbelief at the menu prices. Once we got her to focus on the description, not the cost, even she settled in to enjoy the gourmet feasts. Nightly, we returned to our comfortable beds well sated and eager for the next day of R&R.

We couldn't have asked for better weather: Not too hot, not too cool... juuuuust right! Even the jellyfish that invaded Waikiki Beach for three days during our stay, stinging hundreds, stayed away from us. Side trips to Pearl Harbor (somber and made us all think of my dad who served in the South Pacific) and a Diamond Head hike for Meaghan, Barry, and Michael were the only alternative activities to vegging out on our loungers. It was truly a glorious, fun-filled, relaxing time, absent of any major seizure episodes. The most complicating aspect of the trip was ensuring Michael was hand-checked through security since he had a pacemaker. Michael was relaxing after multiple years of force-fed education. The rest of us were relaxed just knowing life, at least in one sense, would be easier for him. Again, we were creeping toward a state of hopefulness regarding the potential of success of the VNS. For a brief moment in time, we were indeed viewing the world through pink-tinted glasses and enjoying what we saw. Mahalo!

"I think we're here for each other." —*Carol Burnett*

Marking Time

The days in the Connolly household were definitely different in the fall of 2003. Our graduates were both living at home and re-adjusting to sharing a bathroom and household chores. Meaghan was working in my friend Suzanne's pediatric practice following her acceptance to law school that would begin in January. Michael kept busy by going to Madeline's several days a week, and for the first time in his life, he was reading recreationally. It was an indescribably wonderful feeling to know he was actually enjoying the written word, AND he didn't have to worry about a test on the material!

I was able to manage my sporadic work-related trips because Meaghan's schedule was flexible. During one two-week span where my work location was only two freeway exits away, Michael managed on his own. He hadn't had a daytime seizure in quite some time but the fear of one occurring when no one else was around still had a grip on me. In addition, he did have a tendency to nap in the afternoon and he was still having seizures during sleep which could escalate if he didn't swipe his VNS with the magnetic device. However cluttered my mind was with the pessimistic "what ifs," Michael seemed to relish the time on his own and felt, I'm sure, a speck of independence and freedom.

By the time the holiday season arrived, Michael was already beginning to talk about summer courses he could take at the community college. I was somewhat wary since the titration of his meds downward was a very slow process, and he wasn't as alert as we had anticipated, in response to the VNS. We were aware we needed to be patient. Progress, however slow, was occurring in the right direction. I came to accept, with Madeline's assistance, that it wasn't the time that it would take to get there that mattered; it was the eventual outcome of independence for our son that was the goal. Both Barry and I felt at the time that the goal was achievable if certain steps occurred along the way: better seizure control, reduction in medications, internalization of learning techniques, and VNS success.

The holiday season consisted of the usual: my mom arrived about a week before Christmas, just in time to celebrate her birthday, and Gerry arrived the day before Christmas Eve. Gerry brought along his new girlfriend, Suzanne. Christmas Eve was, as always, a boisterous co-mingling of family, neighbors, and friends.

We ended up extending my mom's visit by two weeks when blizzard conditions from the Midwest to the East Coast on the day of her departure, made the prospect of arriving on time and in the intended destination city, pretty shaky. I was glad. I hadn't worked much and was getting pretty used to her presence in the house. Since she was staying, she'd be able to attend the Buick Invitational Golf Tournament with Meaghan and me. Plus, she'd also be around for our Superbowl party. The golf was great fun—John Daly's first win in a long time. Mom was rooting heartily for him in the eighteenth green bleachers. He'd signed her baseball cap with a green sharpie the year before, reaching for it over many other outstretched hands. Yep, he had a true blue fan in Mary Sullivan. The Superbowl was great, too. Mom's New England Patriots claimed another title. Per our routine, our friend Tom ran the football squares board, and, as usual, some non-football-focused female guest ran away with most of the pool money.

The day finally came when my mom left, and as with all her departures, it took a few days to adjust to passing by the guestroom in the morning and not seeing her white head peeking from under the covers.

By spring, Meaghan had a couple of months of law school under her belt. She was always reading and preparing for class, emerging from her room for meals and an occasional TV show. She had weathered the dreaded law school practice of being called upon in all her classes. Her confidence was growing with each completed course. We were pretty confident, even so early on, that she had found her niche. Michael, not surprisingly, was becoming bored with hanging around and stepped up his quest to take some summer courses. He decided on three adult-ed courses; two were computer related and one was a sketch course.

Springtime means baseball, and in our household, that meant the start of the Padre season in their new ballpark, Petco. We really enjoyed our twenty plus games seated in the sixth row just behind third base and Meaghan's favorite Padre, Sean Burroughs. The team didn't do well enough to get anywhere in the post season, but the sunshine, family camaraderie, and love of the game, helped the spring and summer months pass pleasantly. And to cap it all off, the baseball season ended spectacularly with our beloved Red Sox FINALLY capturing the World Series. The hooting, hollering, and plain old screeching emanating from our house during the Yankees play-off series was not to be believed. Michael likes to relay what our next door neighbor Kevin said, "How could two little women make so much noise?"

Since a year earlier, we had experienced our special tropical vacation in Oahu, we decided a city trip should be this summer's travel experience. Where better than New York City? I was happy to learn that the new no-frills airline Jet Blue was flying direct from San Diego to New York City for a very reasonable fare. Why not try the new kid on the block with the sassy attitude and individual Direct TVs for all seats? I booked our flights. I frequented the travel books and Internet and found a two-bedroom suite-like room in what I thought was a good location, for under $300 per night. Though later, I was not excessively happy with our Thirty-fifth Avenue location across from the Empire State Building and little else; the place was clean, functional, and ensured us plenty of exercise. We followed a frenetic pace for seven days of sightseeing, Broadway shows (fabulous *Hairspray* and hilarious *Producers*), and one of our favorite activities, sampling some of the world's best restaurants.

We conducted a pizza tasting over the course of several days' lunches. The Connolly's concluded that John's, Angelo's, and Lombardi's were all great and if pressed, we'd rank them in that order. We also determined that we can get better New York Deli in San Diego than what we experienced at one of the more renowned NYC deli locations. However, we know there is no chance of replicating our experience at Mario Batali's Babbo in Greenwich Village where Michael had the "best calamari ever" and we dined on delicacies such as sweetbreads, beef cheeks, garbanzo bean bruschetta, and ground lamb served in mint "envelopes." THAT was a memorable evening. We visited my cousin Meg and her husband Mike in their hip Tribeca loft and dined with them at trendy 66, where incredibly delicious Chinese specialties were served to us from a chrome lazy susan. We definitely felt we had landed in one of the "in" spots. Our final favorite dining experience was Tribeca's Nobu where we enjoyed delightful Japanese cuisine but Meaghan and I were quite sad that we failed to have a Robert DeNiro sighting.

One morning, the boys and girls split up. Michael and Barry went to the Empire State Building (too high for us) and Meaghan and I went to the *Today* show (too early and too hokey for the guys). Barry and Michael truly enjoyed the panoramic views of the city and took plenty of pictures for us. Meaghan and I were happy to see the perky and quite cute Katie and handsome Matt, but were disappointed Al was not in town. We were a little unsettled by the screechers—"I LOVE you, Katie! Please come HERE, Katie! You're my idol, Katie!" and so on. After we got our mugs on camera for one-tenth of a second, we left for the quieter activity of seeking a knock-off purse from the unauthorized vendors traveling with their blanketed shopping carts around Rockefeller Center.

We met my high school friend, Toni, one day for lunch and she toured us through Ground Zero and St. Paul's Chapel across the street. It was a sobering experience and it re-affirmed a philosophy of making the most of each day we have on this earth.

The frenzied cab rides were balanced by moments of peace and serenity within St. Patrick's. The concrete sidewalks and skyscrapers that felt almost claustrophobic to me while we were among them, took on beautiful hues and created a majestic panorama when viewed from the surrounding waterways of our tourist ferry.

It was a great trip. Michael was amused by the plays, enthused about the food, and seemed to thoroughly enjoy the hustle and bustle of the city. We had late nights, early risings, busy days and blessedly, no seizures. Imagine… the spirit of mahalo in New York City!

"Life is in the here and now, not in the there and afterwards. This day, with all the travail and joy that it brings to our doorstep, is the expression of eternal life. Either we meet it, we live it—or we miss it." —*Vimala Thakar*

Leap of Fate

Michael's experience taking non-credit courses on campus at the community college during the summer of 2004, went well. He became better versed in finding his way around Windows software and it seemed as though he gained some dexterity and depth perception in his art class. He was diligent in completing his assignments and he seemed to be enjoying the learning process. He was anxious though, to begin some formal classes.

In consultation with Madeline, Michael, and his coaches at Falcone Institute, we decided Michael should take two online courses for credit in the fall. Depending on the outcome, he could take at least one class on campus the following semester. Michael chose an English History course and a course about becoming a master student. They were far more work than I had anticipated; requiring three times weekly discussion board postings in addition to reading assignments, projects, and tests. Michael met with his coach for three sessions each week and worked independently the other days. Over the course of the semester, his requests for assistance at home decreased to "none needed." He still became somewhat overwhelmed with testing, but managed to do quite well if he practiced the relaxation techniques taught by his coaches and Madeline. He was still nervous and uncomfortable meeting new people in new situations, but he managed to do both as one of his assignments (overcome your worst fear) during the Epilepsy Foundation holiday fundraiser. He received Bs in both courses; testimony to his persistence and commitment. He was quite pleased with himself and we were very proud of his accomplishment, not just in attaining good grades but in making some real effort to expand his personal horizons and overcome some of his fears.

Michael had been under the care of Dr. Tecoma since his nineteenth birthday when insurance coverage for a Children's Hospital practitioner ceased. Dr. Tecoma had patiently titrated several medications downward and adjusted Michael's VNS about every three months. It was a slow process but when Dr. Nespeca remarked on Michael's heightened state of alertness at Gingerbread City, the holiday fundraiser, "Wow, Michael's much more alert than when I took care of him", it was yet another reliable indicator that positive change was occurring.

VNS and medication changes were not the only measures used to enhance Michael's health. I attributed some of Michael's increased well being to regular gym workouts and exercise, which added some muscle to his frame and improved his endurance (however reluctant and resistant he was to the process). A reasonably healthy but non-restrictive diet increased his weight and gave him freedom of choice in one aspect of his life. Another addition to Michael's fitness and health regimen during the year was chiropractic care, which resulted in greatly improved posture and carriage. And, the usual suspects of vitamins and antioxidants continued to be taken daily along with prescription meds. Michael was definitely looking good and feeling better; physically and emotionally.

Meaghan completed her first year of law school in December. Though she didn't know what particular field of law she wanted to practice, she was undoubtedly on the right career track. She seemed to enjoy living at home again, and, of course, we were delighted with the arrangement. We felt we had much to celebrate during the upcoming holidays.

For this year's visit, my mother PLANNED a two-month stay. She arrived the day before her birthday and rested from the cross-country trip. On the 17th, we took her to The Marine Room, wherein she pronounced her lamb chops "the best anywhere" and proceeded to begin her seventy-eighth year with vigor and appearance belying her years.

Gerry visited too, but this year, due to a messy mid-year split, he was without Suzanne. He seemed unusually happy though, and we all suspected that Suzanne was in his life again. He mentioned her name a few times and spent quite a lot of cell phone time in the backyard. In addition, he had adopted a dog from the pound in October or November. That move simply did not seem compatible with his heavy out-of-town travel schedule. SOMEONE was watching that dog. We didn't know if we should be happy or not given the history of their previous relationship, so we settled for a time on just not reacting or asking and trying to enjoy another Christmas season with one another.

On Christmas Eve, the house was as packed as ever and two large stockpots of duck gumbo were consumed. I had been after Barry for years to add a third pot. "If the Christensen boys had been around this year, there wouldn't have been enough," I argued. I fretted about the small stuff: the ham from the butcher's was definitely NOT up to the quality of the spiral-cut store brand, the turkey was dry, and I should have arranged the food differently to encourage people to mingle more. I vowed I would do things differently next year. What a thrill to have such trivial worries!

We closed out our third year in a row at the home of the Wertzberger's. Rory, their daughter, has been a friend of Meaghan's since the family moved from New Jersey during the girls' grammar school years. The older Wertzberger girls, Reagan and Jessica, son, Max, and parents, Ina and Stuart, have always attended our Christmas Eve celebration. So, in an effort to continue the holiday spirit beyond Christmas, Ina started her own gathering of an eclectic group to ring in the New Year "California style," that is, from 6:00 to 9:00 p.m. Now, each December 31, the Connollys, Wertzbergers, Mary Sullivan, and assorted other changing guests, gather in the coziness of Ina and Stuart's home and dine on chicken marabella from the pages of the Silver Palate cookbook. This time we bade farewell rather fondly to 2004, a remarkable year without crisis or drama. May there be many more like it!

My breathing was shallow, my stomach was full of butterflies, my heart was pattering away, but I was SURE not to show any of it as I dropped Michael off to attend his first official on-campus class at the local community college in January. As I drove away watching him disappear in my rearview mirror, my eyes filled as I felt excitement, fear and anxiety, pride and hope. My goodness, I realized, I felt much like I had when I left Meaghan and Michael at school their first day of kindergarten! I was nervous about the anonymity of a college campus. But, this step simply had to be taken. I would do something to occupy myself and not let my fears get the best of me. Hours later, there he was at the pick-up area...my handsome, smiling, junior college student.

The events of early 2005 led to some interesting discussions around the kitchen table. Michael's queries about the Schiavo debacle, the use of steroids in baseball, the election of the Pope, and even about the "runaway bride," were indicators he was listening: to the news and to conversations. It has become routine to observe him paging through magazines, books, and on a nightly basis; my cookbooks, noting from his perch on the kitchen counter what Mario Batali recipe I should attempt next. He's even expressed interest in pursuing some culinary arts courses. Once oblivious to other people's reactions and body language, Michael is taking cues and in many instances, thoughtfully forming his words and opinions. He isn't always on the mark but he is engaging in the world around him. We are not witnessing remarkable, dramatic moments. Instead, we are observing a series of subtle, sweet, baby steps of progress.

And now...it's spring again. There was another Buick Open. Tiger won. There was another Superbowl. New England won again. My mother made it to Ireland and back for the tenth time. Meaghan's halfway through law school. Jessica's having a baby. Katharine Tremblay is home. Gerry's back with Suzanne. And...slowly, deliberately, and sometimes surely, Michael is finding his way.

My friend Nancy wondered, "How can you end the book? Your story isn't over."

I have no illusions. I do not know how all this will turn out. I know only that spring will turn to summer, summer to fall, fall to winter, and then— the promises of spring will return again. Hope, after all, springs eternal.

About the Author

Mary Lou Connolly, a registered nurse with over thirty years of health care experience, has authored many articles for publication in nursing and home health care journals. She has appeared on the series *Frontline* in a story about health insurance coverage, and she has testified before a congressional committee about the positive effects of home health care. She routinely speaks to professional audiences about health care issues, and she has spoken before a number of community groups about epilepsy. She is a member of the Board of Directors of the Epilepsy Foundation of San Diego County. None of the author's health care experiences or professional achievements prepared her to be the mother of a child with a serious chronic illness. It was, she notes, a "learn as you go" experience. She has shared her story because of a desire to increase public awareness and understanding about living with epilepsy. Mary Lou lives with her husband Barry and children Meaghan and Michael, in Del Mar, California.